WALKING YOUR WAY TO VITALITY

Praise for *Walking Your Way to Vitality*

"This book is an amazing resource for anyone wishing to improve their health and well-being just by walking! The authors provide us with clear, accessible instructions and videos to create an individualized walking routine based on the wisdom of Traditional Chinese Medicine. The historical and scientific introductions to each of the 'walks' emphasize the importance of the breath and the focus of the mind, as well as the specific body movements. From power walks to meditative circle walks, these practices can help the mind, body, and spirit across the lifespan. While I can't wait to have this as a resource for my adult patients, I'd love to see these self-care practices taught in our school system to young children as well!"

—**Kirsten Tillisch**, MD, professor of medicine,
David Geffen School of Medicine at UCLA

"Movement is one of the five pillars of health, and walking is one of the most basic forms of exercise for human beings. If you love walking or are looking to add it to your routine, you will love this book. Dr. Jacques MoraMarco and Dr. Yun Kim have outlined the different styles of walking to maximize your health and longevity. In addition, each style focuses on a different aspect of your physical, spiritual, and emotional well-being. Integrating the different styles will keep your walking routine fresh and invigorating."

—**Rick Csintalan**, MD, chief,
Department of Orthopedic Surgery, Kaiser Permanente

"An enlightening approach to walking that transforms a simple daily activity into a profound practice for health and longevity. This book brilliantly bridges ancient Eastern wisdom with modern wellness, offering readers practical tools to enhance their vitality with every step."

—**Sanghoon Lee**, MD (Korean Medicine),
PhD, MPH, MBA, DiplOM, LAc; director, International
Education Institute of Korean Medicine, Kyung Hee University;
and deputy director, East-West Medical Research Institute,
WHO Collaborating Center for Traditional Medicine

"Dr. MoraMarco has long been a source of inspiration in both my personal and professional journey. In *Walking Your Way to Vitality*, he distills decades of wisdom into a practice that reconnects us with the simplest, most powerful tools for well-being—our breath, our body, and our awareness. This book is more than a guide to walking; it's a gentle invitation to return to presence and vitality in every step."

—**Brian Call**, US Navy Seal

"As a practitioner of meditation and yoga for over 50 years, I highly recommend mindful walking as an essential part of one's daily life. I urge you to incorporate these practices, aligning mind, body, and heart, and you will be happy."

—**Bong Dal Kim**, OMD, LAc, founder,
Emperor's College of Traditional Medicine

WALKING YOUR WAY TO VITALITY

Integrating Walking, Breathwork, and Mindfulness Into Your Daily Exercise

Jacques MoraMarco, OMD, DAOM, LAc
and Yun Kim, EdD, DAOM, LAc

Skyhorse Publishing

Photos by Wil Fernandez @ffcinema_

Skyhorse Publishing books may be purchased in bulk at special discounts for sales promotion, corporate gifts, fund-raising, or educational purposes. Special editions can also be created to specifications. For details, contact the Special Sales Department, Skyhorse Publishing, 307 Fifth Avenue, 4th Floor, New York, NY 10016 or info@skyhorsepublishing.com.

Skyhorse® and Skyhorse Publishing® are registered trademarks of Skyhorse Publishing, Inc.®, a Delaware corporation.

Visit our website at www.skyhorsepublishing.com.

Please follow our publisher Tony Lyons on Instagram @tonylyonsisuncertain.

10 9 8 7 6 5 4 3 2 1

Library of Congress Cataloging-in-Publication Data is available on file.

Cover design by David Ter-Avanesyan
Cover illustration by Shutterstock

Print ISBN: 978-1-5107-8471-0
Ebook ISBN: 978-1-5107-8472-7

Printed in the United States of America

To all of our students. May you have health, vitality, and eternal spring.

Contents

Superior physicians do not cure diseases. They prevent diseases. Treating a disease after it has arisen is like digging a well when one is thirsty or casting weapons when the battle has begun. It is too late.

—The Yellow Emperor's Classic of Internal Medicine

Introduction

Running water is never stale and a door-hinge never gets worm-eaten. So it is with a person's physique and vital energy.

—Sun Simiao

If you are passionate about walking and manage to walk every day, this book is for you. In it, you will find truly new insights and practical tips about how to maximize the health benefits of your daily walk. But if you walk as exercise only occasionally or have not done a lot of walking in the past, this book is also for you.

In these pages, you will learn why walking is among the most important forms of exercise you can perform to improve your physical, mental, and emotional health. You will find that walking does not need to be strenuous or boring.

If you are like most people, your method of walking is the fundamental "one foot in front of the other" style, whether you are going just a half mile around your block or pursuing the goal of 10,000 steps per day. We call that the "traditional" walk, as it is what comes naturally to humans. You step outside and just start walking, perhaps listening to a podcast or just taking in your neighborhood. However you do it, you are just walking.

This book teaches you that this traditional walking style can be much more varied, interesting, and fun. We will teach you five additional walking styles that are not like the traditional walk. These styles can be used alone or in combination with the traditional walk or with each other to maximize your benefits. Using these five styles, you can transform your traditional walk into a different experience each day.

"Wait," you are thinking, "there are other walking styles?"

Yes, there are. Like dancing, there are many ways to move your arms and legs as well as to incorporate breath patterns when you walk. We are not talking about power walking or speed walking, but about literally five other very different styles of walking that you likely had no idea existed.

The styles we teach in this book are largely derived from ancient East Asian concepts of bodily energy and health, called *qi* (from China, pronounced as "chi") and from the concept of *prana* (from India, meaning life force). Maintaining one's qi or prana was (and still is today) perceived as the source of vitality, good health, and longevity. As such, many physical exercises, often combined with breathing patterns, were developed to support one's vital energy. The practices of tai chi, qigong, and many forms of yoga have their foundation in these concepts. These movements are rooted in thousands of years of East Asian healing methods that target improving lung, liver, heart, kidney, and stomach function, maintaining strength and balance, reducing stress, and calming the mind. In addition, some elements of the five walking styles we teach are also based on the practice of mindfulness meditation and East Asian spiritual practices. One walking style incorporates the breath patterns used by people who live at high altitudes in the Himalayas.

We will begin in week 1 with a discussion of the basic "traditional" style of walking, with a goal to clarify many common questions about the traditional walk, such as:

- How many steps should I strive for: 4,000? 6,000? 8,000? 10,000?

- Do I get extra health benefits by walking more than 10,000 steps?
- What is power walking and is it worth doing?
- How fast should I walk?
- Should I decrease the number of steps I aim to walk as I age?
- Do I need to use a smartwatch to track my steps and heart rate?
- Should I warm up before walking?
- Are there any risks in walking?
- Does walking backward offer benefits?
- And more.

Following this chapter for week 1, each of the next chapters will introduce you to one of the other walking styles we want to teach you:

- **Week 2:** The Vitality Walk for Energy
- **Week 3:** The Mindfulness Walk for Inner Calm
- **Week 4:** The Immune Power Walk to Regain Health
- **Week 5:** The Tai Chi Animal Walks for Balance
- **Week 6:** The Circle Walk for Self-Reflection
- **Week 7:** Integrating the Walks and Staying Motivated

Each chapter will describe the origins of the walk and the health benefits that style of walking brings you. We will then explain how to do the walking style with easy-to-follow directions. But just as it can be difficult to teach someone a dance routine using just words, we know that the written explanations cannot explain everything. Thus, in each chapter, we are providing photos that show the positions, as well as a QR code that links to online videos where you can see the walks being performed in detail—the exact movements of the arms and/or legs and the coordination with the breath if necessary.

By the end of the book, you will have learned five incredibly healthful walking styles that can make your daily walk more interesting and fun. We suggest that you learn one walk per week and then begin integrating it into your daily walking schedule. Some of the five walks can be done alone, replacing your daily walk. But most of them are walking styles you can integrate into the time you spend on your daily walk. For example, if you walk for thirty minutes, you can spend ten minutes of that time doing one of the walks such as the Vitality Walk or the Immune Power Walk.

Ultimately, over the course of five weeks, you will learn about these five new walks and be able to choose using them individually or combining them in different ways to create a completely new walking experience each day.

About Us

We write this book based on decades of experience in studying and teaching East Asian medicine. We are also avid walkers and practice these walking styles in our daily lives.

Jacques MoraMarco is the dean emeritus at the former Emperor's College of Traditional East Asian Medicine. During his career at the school, he supervised doctoral students who provided acupuncture in the post-traumatic stress disorder (PTSD) clinic at the VA Greater Los Angeles Health System. A licensed acupuncturist since 1977, he took the first acupuncture licensing examination ever administered in the state of California. He apprenticed with See Han Kim, a renowned teacher of traditional Korean medicine, who was trained monastically. He completed his postgraduate work at Ecole Européene d'Acupuncture in Paris. From 1994 to 2004, he studied Sun tai chi with Sun Shurong in Beijing, China, and he is a fourth-generation lineage holder of Sun Tai Chi. He is a cofounder of the International Sun Tai Chi Association.

Yun Kim is the founder of Emperor's Wellness, a doctor of traditional East Asian medicine, and a fifth-generation lineage holder of Sun tai chi, and has practiced mindful meditation for the past twenty years, learning from the renowned teachers Thich Nhat Hanh and Trudy Goodman. A licensed acupuncturist in the state of California, she completed her doctoral clinical rotation at the PTSD clinic at the VA Greater Los Angeles Health System and maintains an acupuncture practice in Los Angeles. She earned her Doctor of Education at the USC [University of Southern California] Rossier School of Education.

Together, we are well versed in East Asian medical practices and know the importance of maintaining vitality and good health through walking, breathing, and mindfulness meditation. We hope that you will incorporate these principles and practices in your daily practice, nourish your mind and body, and enhance the quality of your life.

Week 1
The Traditional Daily Walk

A good traveler has no fixed plans and is not intent on arriving.

—Lao Tzu

Walking is increasingly recognized as one of the easiest and most healthy activities one can do at any age. Its popularity is growing in every demographic, from Gen Zs all the way to the baby boomers. In neighborhoods across the US, people are forming walking clubs—or even getting a dog so they have a reason to go for a daily walk. Walking is the most popular exercise in the US; according to the 2022 National Health Interview Survey, in a sampling of US households, almost one in six adults had taken a walk for leisure in the past week.

The human form was made for walking. Our genes are encoded with a drive to crawl, then to stand up and walk. We have developed all sorts of modes of transportation, from subways and buses to cars, trains, and planes, all in an effort to make our lives easier, faster, and more interesting. Most of us can find also great pleasure in taking a simple walk around our neighborhood or in parks, on beaches, or in the mountains.

We are increasingly discovering both that walking imparts huge health benefits—and that the converse is true. If we do not walk, we could pay a heavy price for neglecting our human imperative. The truth is, the human body needs regular walking to stay healthy and fit.

Walking has many critical health benefits that have been scientifically proven in hundreds of studies over the last eighty years. Consider some of the scientific research that has been done to investigate the advantages of walking:

- **Walking lowers your risk of heart disease, the leading cause of death in the US**. According to the American Heart Association's *2025 Heart Disease and Stroke Statistics Update*, heart disease remains the leading cause of death in the US.[1] Cardiovascular diseases, including heart disease and stroke, claim more lives in the US than all forms of cancer and accidental deaths combined. The risk factors for heart disease include high blood pressure and obesity, which continue to grow at alarming rates. Nearly 47 percent of US adults have high blood pressure and more than 72 percent of US adults have unhealthy weight (currently defined as body mass index ≥25, with nearly 42 percent having obesity (currently defined as body mass index ≥30).

Many studies have confirmed that a little walking goes a long way in strengthening the heart by increasing blood circulation to heart tissue. A Harvard Health report published in 2017 concluded that about twenty-one minutes per day can reduce the risk of heart attack by 30 percent.[2] Another study, published in the *European Journal of Preventive Cardiology* in 2023, found that walking just 2,337 steps a day reduced the risk of dying from diseases of the heart and blood vessels.[3] Furthermore, an analysis of 226,889 people from seventeen different studies around the world indicated that the more you walk, the greater the health benefits. In those studies, it was shown that the risk of dying from any cause or from cardiovascular disease decreases significantly with every 500 to 1,000 extra steps you walk.[4] Another study published in March 2025 in *the British Journal of Sports Medicine* suggested that any amount of daily steps above 2,200 was associated with a reduced risk of death from cardiovascular disease.[5]

The upshot is that people who walk have significantly lower rates of coronary disease and heart attack than people who do not exercise. The reason for this difference is worth understanding. First, exercise improves circulation, which increases the blood volume and oxygen-carrying capacity. This nourishes the heart tissue cells. The increased circulation also lowers blood fats and increases the high-density lipoproteins (HDLs, or the "good cholesterol" elements in our blood that help protect against heart disease). Increased circulation also strengthens and expands the size of the heart's blood vessels, which helps clean out fatty deposits that can block blood flow and cause heart attacks. Finally, the increased circulation helps the heart develop a lower resting heart rate, so that it is less taxed during normal activities.

- **Walking promotes better circulation throughout the entire body.** With better blood flow, all the body tissues experience increased oxygenation. The same positive effects in the blood vessels of the heart occur in the blood vessels of the lungs, legs, and brain. The entire body thus benefits from the fresh oxygen and nutrients supplied to tissues and from the cleansing of fat deposits on arterial walls.

Walking especially helps the legs, because when leg muscles are exercised, they are able to more forcefully push the blood against gravity through the veins back up to the heart. This contributes to lower blood pressure (since the heart does not need to work as hard to force blood to be returned to it), and it reduces the chances of stroke from blood clots that often begin in the legs when people are sedentary.

- **Walking reduces the risk of cancer.** Cancer is the second leading cause of death in the US, causing one in every six deaths. According to the American Cancer Society (ACS), one in three adult men and women will develop cancer at some time in their lives, and one in six will die from it. For men, the most common sites of cancer are prostate, lungs, and colorectal; for women, they are breast, lung, and colorectal.

Diet and smoking are responsible for a large percentage of cancer cases, but a third factor identified by the ACS is lack of exercise. Meanwhile, studies have found that walking can lower the risk of developing cancer. In a study of 140,000 people conducted by the ASC, researchers found that even low levels of walking are linked with lower mortality. As a result, the ACS recommends that adults get at least 150 minutes of moderate-intensity activity, such as a brisk walk (a pace of three miles per hour) each week spread throughout the week. But the study even showed that participants who walked fewer than two hours per week had a lower death risk than participants who did not walk at all.[6]

- **Walking lowers the likelihood of developing type 2 diabetes.** The cause of type 2 diabetes remains unclear, but research has shown that diet and exercise play key roles in preventing it or helping to mitigate high blood sugar. Complications from diabetes can be serious and include infections, kidney disease, blindness, and amputations. It is estimated that one in three adults in the US has prediabetes (meaning high blood sugar), and one in ten adults has full-blown type 2 diabetes.

The American Diabetes Association indicates that walking has many health benefits that help prevent developing type 2 diabetes. For instance, walking has beneficial effects on the pancreas, which is the key to keeping your blood sugar in check. Research has shown that walking improves how fast glucose is absorbed from the bloodstream into muscle cells, thus minimizing the potential for type 2 diabetes. The American Diabetes Association endorses walking, as it lowers blood glucose (blood sugar) levels, increases insulin sensitivity and metabolism, and helps with weight loss or maintenance.

- **Walking lowers the risk of osteoporosis.** Osteoporosis is a condition in which the bones have less mass and are more porous, making them more susceptible to breaking, especially in the hip and spine. Often the person with the disease is not aware of it until a fall causes a bone fracture. Among the risk factors for osteoporosis are low calcium intake and a lack of physical activity. According to the National Osteoporosis Foundation, over 10 million Americans have osteoporosis, and another 44 million have such low bone mass that they are at risk of the disease. About 80 percent of these people are women. The

Mayo Clinic recommends that low-impact forms of exercise such as walking are best to lower the risk of injuries for those who have osteoporosis. Walking strengthens both muscles and bones, and several of the walking routines in this book improve your flexibility and your balance, reducing the risks of tripping and falling.

- **Walking strengthens muscles and aids in joint stabilization.** As we get older, we need to continue to exercise in order to keep our muscles active, especially in the legs, and our joints strong. If we don't, we will move through our days stiff, inflexible, and uncomfortable. Walking is a great way to stay strong without risking the injuries that come with vigorous, high-impact exercise.

- **Walking improves lung capacity.** When you are involved in a physical activity such as walking, your oxygen uptake is increased. That's because walking strengthens the muscles of the chest and diaphragm. This makes more oxygen available to nourish all the systems of your body.

- **Walking helps manage your weight.** Walking is generally far more effective than dieting or fasting.

Though we don't advocate counting calories, it might be interesting to note as a reference point in our fitness program that walking consumes between roughly two hundred and four hundred calories per hour, depending on the pace. More importantly, after walking, our body's metabolism continues to work at a higher rate as well. Since it takes 3,500 calories to lose a pound, this means that if you walk five hours per week at a moderate pace (three miles per hour) and burn 350 calories per hour, you can lose one pound in two weeks. This type of slow weight loss is the healthiest and most likely not to reverse. It may seem like a small amount of weight to lose, but the fact is, the average person can easily lose twenty-five to thirty pounds in one year—without even a diet change—through a simple walking program of five hours per week.

- **Walking tones muscles, improves the mobility of our joints, and helps prevent loss of bone mass and bone fractures**. Even if you have arthritis, walking can be beneficial in reducing joint pain and stiffness. If you have back pain, walking is an excellent low-impact exercise that helps increase blood circulation to help heal spinal inflammation.

- **Walking can help mitigate overeating**, which is perhaps the most common reason people gain weight, other than genetic factors. Obviously, walking also helps you tone and strengthen your muscles, while burning the fat that our body stores around stagnant muscle areas.

- **Walking is an effective stress reliever**, not just from a psychological point of view, but also from a biological one. This is because exercise increases the level of the chemicals in the brain known as endorphins and neuropeptides. Scientists have known for years that higher levels of endorphins (which include enkephalins, beta-endorphin, and dynorphin) and neuropeptides (such as dopamine) in the brain lead to mood elevation and an increased sense of calm and well-being. In contrast, lower levels of endorphins and neuropeptides can lead to fatigue, depression, loss of motivation, and many chronic conditions. Combined, all of these physiological factors help to create a sense of well-being, which further helps you relax your entire body.

- **Walking improves thought clarity, memory, and concentration.** The increased oxygen supply in the brain due to walking helps with thinking more clearly.

- **Walking can reduce risk of developing Alzheimer's and dementia.** A study done at the University of Calgary in Alberta, Canada that tracked nearly three thousand participants between the ages of seventy and seventy-nine indicated that walking daily appears to reduce the risk of cognitive decline due to Alzheimer's, especially among people who have a genetic predisposition for the disease. Participants who maintained or increased their walking habits over the years of the study showed greater improvements in mental processing speed and executive function.[7] In addition, according to a study published in a 2022 issue of *JAMA Neurology* involving over seventy-eight thousand participants, people between the ages of forty and seventy-nine who took approximately 3,800 steps a day at any speed cut their risk of dementia by 25 percent, and people who walked as much as 9,826 steps per day were 50 percent less likely to develop dementia within seven years. The same study also found that people who walked with "purpose" at a pace over forty steps a minute were able to cut their risk of dementia by 57 percent with just 6,315 steps a day.[8]

- **Walking helps you age more slowly.** Because it increases the oxygen supply to all cells in the body, walking keeps the lung and heart tissues resilient and improves muscle mass. Although scientists do not yet fully understand aging, it is known that reduced oxygenation, the natural loss of resiliency in the lung and heart tissues, and the slow loss of muscle mass all contribute to aging more quickly. Between the ages of thirty-five and fifty, in fact, the body loses muscle mass at the rate of one to 5 percent per decade, and after the age of thirty, the heart loses its ability to pump by about 6 to 8 percent per decade. This is why sedentary people who do not rejuvenate these losses through exercise have five times (yes, five times!) the risk of heart disease as those who engage in regular physical activity.[9]

  Research has shown, however, some forms of mindfulness meditation can prevent telomere shortening or even lengthen telomeres, thus contributing to better brain health and the possibility of a longer life. Telomeres are the protective caps at the ends of chromosomes. Over time, when our cells divide, the telomeres get shorter. Eventually, if they become too short, the ends of the chromosomes can fray or stick to each other. This process is believed to be an element in the causation of cancer as well as an accelerator of aging.

All in all, there is absolutely no doubt about the health benefits of walking. Indeed, walking is now the exercise of choice and highly recommended by leading medical institutions and doctors. It is regularly prescribed for severe heart attack patients and for people coming out of nearly every type of surgery, compared to the early twentieth century when doctors prescribed weeks of bed rest. Movement gets the circulatory system back in shape, rebuilds heart tissue, tones muscles, and contributes to positive mental health which, in turn, aids the recuperation process.

The Passion of a Daily Walk

We hope this explanation of the tremendous health benefits of walking inspires and motivates you to take a daily walk, or at least to walk several days a week. If you already have a walking routine, congratulations. You are likely aware of how much a daily walk improves your life and you can see the results. If you do not yet have a commitment to a daily routine of walking, now is the time to make a promise to begin doing so.

Keep in mind that the traditional daily walk—one foot in front of the other—can be as varied as the environment and climate you live in. You can walk somewhere in your neighborhood that is flat and easy, or you can go somewhere with a mix of flat areas and hills. You can walk in the early morning at sunrise, after lunch, or in the evening at sunset. You can drive to a nearby park or a beach area. You can walk in the sunshine or even in the rain. You can walk alone, with a partner or family member, or join a group of walkers who meet on weekends for a jaunt. Whenever you walk, you can calm your nerves from stress. We'll talk more about getting and staying motivated to walk later in the book.

Answers to Common Questions about Walking

One might think that the traditional walk is pretty straightforward, but in recent years, a wide assortment of questions has appeared that seems to have created a lot of confusion. In this section, we want to address these common questions and add to your knowledge about walking.

How Many Steps per Day?

The first question that nearly every walker has is just how many steps are the right number to strive for during a walk to get real health benefits? Is it 4,000, 6,000, 8,000, or even 10,000? Many people have come to believe 10,000 steps is the correct answer, but this appears to be based on a marketing gimmick. In 1965, a Japanese company manufactured a wearable device to count steps and named it "Manpokei," which translates into "10,000 steps meter." This brand name took hold and initiated a sort of myth that walkers should strive for 10,000 steps per day to be healthy.

So, is there a more correct number? The best answer to the question is actually "it depends" on a number of factors, including your current physical health, your age, and even your terrain. If you are in good shape, feeling vital and have no health issues, walking 10,000 steps is very doable as your daily goal. If you have a smartphone or smartwatch that tracks your steps, it's easy to set a goal of 10,000 steps and track it. This number of steps converts to roughly five miles, using 2,000 steps per mile as an average (though for people with long strides, 2,000 steps is nearly 2.4 miles). The amount of time you need to walk 10,000 steps is approximately ninety minutes, assuming your pace is about eighteen minutes per 2,000 steps.

For many people, one and half hours of walking time is too much given their stamina or their work and family schedule. If you are still looking for a good workout though, you can aim for 6,000 to 8,000 steps, about three to four miles, which might take you roughly an hour or a bit more.

An interesting research project shows that between 4,400 and 7,500 steps per day is sufficient to lower mortality risk. A study published in the *Journal of the American Medical Association* in May 2019 reported:

> In this cohort study of 16,741 women with a mean age of 72 years, steps per day were measured over 7 days. Women who averaged approximately 4400 steps per day had significantly lower mortality rates during a follow-up of 4.3 years compared with the least active women who took approximately 2700 steps per day; as more steps per day were accrued, mortality rates progressively decreased before leveling at approximately 7500 steps/day.[10]

If you are just starting out to create a daily walking routine, you might begin with a simple goal of 2,000 to 2,500 steps, just to begin building up stamina and a passion for walking. Then, over a period of a few weeks, seek to raise your daily goal incrementally to 4,400 steps, then 5,500, and up to 7,500 if possible, according to your stamina and comfort in walking for longer periods of time.

In general, we believe that the number of steps per day are the most often cited ones, but to be comprehensive, it is worth noting that there are also some statistics showing that one may not need as many steps as the figures cited above. In a 2019 study published in the *British Journal of Sports Medicine*, researchers from the Medical Research Council (MRC) Epidemiology Unit at the University of Cambridge examined research from 196 academic articles reporting on 94 large studies collectively involving more than 30 million participants.[11] Their goal was to identify how much physical activity actually had an effect on the risk of heart disease, cancer, and early death. The results were surprising, suggesting that even fewer than 150 minutes of activity per week, as low as eleven minutes per day, of moderate-intensity activity such as brisk walking reduced the risk of early death by 23 percent, cardiovascular disease by 17 percent, and cancer by 7 percent. While they still recommend that people strive for 150 minutes of moderate-intensity exercise per week (thirty minutes per day, five days per week), they acknowledge that their study proves that even a short workout per day, such as a walk, can have long-term benefits.

In addition to the general guidelines above, the most important recommendation we have is to listen to the body. You may feel absolutely super one day, with lots of energy and stamina. You would thus have no problems spending time walking to reach 8,000 or 10,000 steps. But on another day, you might feel tired or have pain in your foot or leg. Pay attention to these signals indicating that your walk should be shorter, perhaps just 4,000 steps, just fifteen or thirty minutes, no matter how far you go.

Does Age Matter?

In our view, the simple answer to this is "no." In today's world, most people believe that our chronological age is not an indication of our capability to accomplish anything. A few decades ago, it was often said that "sixty was the new fifty," but now many people, recently getting into their retirement years, believe that "seventy is the new sixty."

If you are past the age of eighty (or even seventy or so), the only caveat might be to make sure you feel physically fit to strive for an hour of walking every day. If you begin to feel muscle aches or fatigue, go ahead and skip a day here and there, or decide to walk just three or four days per week.

But the advantage you have in reading this book is that you will gain some alternatives to the traditional daily walk. Several of the five unique walking styles we teach are less strenuous for an older adult, yet still offer significant benefits to stay healthy, fit, and vital.

Treadmill or Outside?

There is a perennial debate about whether the benefits are greater walking on a treadmill rather than outside. Many people have treadmills inside their homes, so the convenience of exercising any time you want is unbeatable for them. Plus, today's sophisticated treadmills offer a variety of programs to customize one's workout to different simulated terrains, and even watch a movie or read a book while you are walking. The cushioned surface of a treadmill provides less impact on joints and feet than a sidewalk, and there's no traffic or other hazards to pose risks to your safety.

On the other hand, walking outdoors provides a more natural experience. Your eyes naturally seek out the horizon line and our bodies relish the sunlight and its warmth. Your senses respond to the fresh air and the feel of the wind on your face and skin. Numerous studies prove that being in nature helps us reduce our stress and relieve us from anxiety and worries. These benefits of walking outside can help us stay motivated to walk every day simply to get relief from being in an office building or our home all day. And of course, if you have a dog, you need to get outside.

Ultimately, the choice is yours. If you own a treadmill or have access to one, you can use time on it to do a cardio workout that is more oriented to raising our heartbeat than a traditional walk might. If you live in a region that has a very harsh, cold climate during some of the year, a treadmill might be the only way to walk every day. But if there is the opportunity to be outdoors, our recommendation is to take advantage of that as often as possible.

How Fast to Walk?

As we discussed in the entry on steps, the average time it takes to walk 2,000 steps (one mile) is about eighteen minutes. This translates into slightly above three miles per hour, which is an average walking speed if you are younger than forty years old. As we age, we do tend to slow down our walking speed.

If you want to do a "brisk" walk, you need to aim for a speed of four miles per hour, thus 2,000 steps in fifteen minutes. Beyond this speed, you are approaching "power walking" or "race walking" which is a specialty type of walking in itself.

These are generalizations, of course, as walking speed depends on many factors such as length of your stride, terrain (flat or hilly), weather (calm or windy, slippery or dry), and other things that can influence your ultimate speed.

If you want to measure your walking speed, you need to time yourself as you walk 100 steps. If you are doing 100 steps per minute, your walking speed is about three miles per hour. Alternatively, you can time yourself as you walk one mile. If your time to do this is twenty minutes, your walking speed is three miles per hour.

On average, a person walking three miles per hour burns about two hundred calories in thirty minutes of walking.

Which Is Better for Our Health: Walking Farther or Faster?

Our view is that this debate can go either way. Each choice has different benefits for your long-term health. This makes deciding which one is best for you a challenge because few people know whether they are at risk for heart disease, cancer, or another condition that might cause an early death. Here's how we might contrast the two:

- Walking longer helps build our endurance and can strengthen our heart and lungs.
- Walking faster also helps our heart as it is a more intense cardio workout. Walking faster also can help burn more calories than walking longer.

Ultimately, either choice is a function of your current conditioning, endurance, and commitment to walking. Both choices can require you to reach beyond your normal capabilities, so it is up to you to decide each day whether you are willing and able to walk faster or farther than you normally do.

Is There Any Value in "Japanese" Walking—the Method of Walking Alternately Fast Then Slow?

Some recent studies have been added to others from decades ago about the benefit of "Japanese" walking, also called "interval walking training" (IWT). Twenty years ago, a study was done showing that middle-aged and older people who alternate between walking fast for three minutes, then slow for three minutes over a total of thirty minutes have lower blood pressure, stronger leg muscles, and higher aerobic capacity than people who walk at a constant moderate pace for thirty minutes. Since that 2007 study, two additional studies—one in 2023 with type 2 diabetics and one in 2024 with people over sixty-five—confirmed that IWT achieved such health benefits as lower cholesterol, lower body mass index (BMI), and greater flexibility.[12]

You might try the Japanese walking style during your traditional walk if you have the energy and stamina for it over thirty minutes. However, many people have difficulty walking fast enough for so long, even when alternating with slow walking, to qualify as IWT, since your pace has to be so rapid that you cannot speak. If you want to try this style of walking, build up to it by starting with alternating fast and slow for just ten or fifteen minutes, then add five more minutes each time you are comfortable at a new plateau of time.

What About Walking Backwards?

You may never have heard of or thought about walking backward (a.k.a. retro-walking), but some experts recommend it for people with back, knee, hip, or ankle problems. In 1915, Patrick Harmon, age fifty, walked backward from San Francisco to New York, supposedly to win a bet. He reported that his ankles had built up a strong sturdiness from the experience.

When you walk backward, it obviously alters the way your feet touch the ground. The ankle hits first, strengthening it. Walking backward also alters which muscles get used in the process, with more emphasis on your glutes, hamstrings, and shins. This is said to help improve your balance, an important health benefit given that falling down is common among people over sixty seventy.

Walking backward also strengthens our glutes and hip flexors, which helps alleviate back pain. It also puts less stress on your joints, especially your knees. This is important for anyone who has arthritis or joint pain or who needs to take precautions to avoid injuries.

There are also brain benefits. Obviously, walking backward is difficult, so it forces the brain to be ever vigilant, coordinating the eyes and feet to avoid obstacles and falls. You must have a heightened level of awareness, paying attention to each step. You cannot walk on automatic pilot, as you can do when walking forward. Due to its counterintuitive nature, backward walking also forces your brain to use different regions than it normally does, related to decision-making and problem solving. This can be very beneficial for people developing cognitive problems or dementia.

Of course, there are risks to walking backward if you do not take enough time to practice it safely. To start, you might try doing it on a treadmill at a very slow walking speed and use the handrails for support. If you start outdoors, you can have someone with you to spot you in case you stumble. You can do it on a pathway you know well so there are no surprise obstacles. Also, it can be wise to alternate between walking forward and backward every minute or so until you are truly comfortable with retro-walking.

How Can I Get and Stay Motivated to Walk?

If you are new to walking on a regular basis, you may find your mind (and body) protesting on some days, convincing you not to go out. This is not unusual when we begin anything new, be it practicing a musical instrument we pledged to learn or committing to read a book a week rather than surfing on our devices. Here are some suggestions to get over those humps in your commitment:

- Take it one day at a time. If your mind tells you, "I cannot possibly do this every day," respond, "Let's go today and enjoy it."

- Start slowly as this chapter recommended, walking ten to fifteen minutes as you build up endurance and begin to appreciate the joy of walking.
- Walk with someone so you are accountable to a partner. Find some topics you enjoy discussing as you walk together.
- Listen to audiobooks or dip into the many excellent podcasts that are available to entertain yourself as you walk. There are even podcast channels for walking.
- Learn a language as you walk, practicing your pronunciation when no one is around to hear.
- Make a list of exercise goals that you truly want to achieve, such as being able to go up a hill in your neighborhood, walking twenty miles per week, or one hundred miles per month.

The Beauty of the Traditional Walk

There is no longer any question that developing a passion for a daily walk (or almost daily) will yield enormous health benefits. You will look better due to the muscle toning, you may maintain your optimal weight, and you will feel less stressed and more focused. Many research studies suggest that you will likely reduce your risks of heart disease, diabetes, dementia, and an early death.

But the point of this book is that there is more to the daily walk than the traditional walking style. In the coming chapters, we will introduce you to five unique styles of walking—each with its own benefits. Practice one of these per week and then integrate it into your traditional daily walk.

Week 2

The Vitality Walk for Energy

In every walk with nature, one receives far more than one seeks.

—John Muir

The traditional walking routine has great health benefits, as you have just seen. But did you know that you can learn a slightly different walking style dedicated to improving your "vitality?" We call it the "Vitality Walk" because it enhances our energy, increases our circulation, improves oxygen flow to every cell in our body, tones the muscles, eliminates fats and toxins from our arteries and veins, and stimulates our mind.

Most of us don't use the word *vitality* much anymore. Think for a moment: how often do you describe yourself or a friend as having tremendous vitality? In all likelihood, not very often.

Vitality refers to having energy and dynamism. It evokes a picture of physical strength and hardiness. For many people, it connotes a sense of youthfulness. If you say that someone has vitality, it is like saying that the person is young and vibrant, regardless of the chronological age.

Isn't vitality a quality you'd like to achieve through walking?

An Ancient Reverence for Vitality

Before we teach the Vitality Walk, it helps to understand the historical perspective that having vitality was the key to preventing weakness, disease, and an early death. In many ancient, traditional cultures, vitality was revered. It implied a wide range of healthful traits, including endurance, longevity, and resistance to illness.

Throughout Asia, vitality was deeply embedded in the worldview of life and health. East Asian medicine is based upon the principle that the human body contains a life force, called qi, which animates all physiological functions in the body. Qi flows along meridians throughout the body, nourishing and rejuvenating all the tissues and organs, including the brain. These meridians are not the same as the nerves or blood vessels, but a separate system of pathways that transport qi energy everywhere.

Qi is essential to good health, because it signifies that a person has the right balance of vital energy flowing through the body. Qi energy promotes good health, both mentally and physically, and helps the body resist disease.

An imbalance of qi causes illness. This occurs because an impediment in the flow of qi to some part of the body weakens a key organ, allowing disease to enter. Caring for an ill person requires figuring out how to restore vitality by rebalancing the qi. To achieve a smooth flowing of qi, one can use acupuncture, acupressure, and herbal treatments, all of which can open up the pathways and restore the proper movement of vital energy.

In the Western world as well, many ancient civilizations also subscribed to a respect for vitality. The code of the ancient Hebrews required them to proactively live a healthy lifestyle to avoid disease. The Book of Leviticus includes instructions on good health and prevention, including paying attention to hygiene, separating the sick from the healthy, and disinfecting clothing and items used by the ill.

Ancient Greek medicine also recognized the connection between maintaining vitality and good health. Based on the theories of the philosopher Empedocles, the early Greek school of medicine (sixth century BCE) believed that the body was composed of good and evil "humors" that had to stay in balance. When the humors were imbalanced, the person became mentally or physically ill. The ancient Greeks admonished citizens to eat well, avoid excesses, and seek out mental and physical harmony in life.

After the ancient Greeks, early Western civilizations likewise emphasized vitality as the most effective preventive medicine for nearly another two thousand years. Because of very slow advances in understanding human anatomy, physiology, and pharmacology, the Greek theory of humors dominated Western medicine throughout the time of the Roman Empire and into the Middle Ages and Renaissance, up until the nineteenth century, when new discoveries about the circulatory system and the proof of germs finally discredited its validity.

Louis Pasteur's late-nineteenth-century discovery that bacteria cause disease is commonly recognized as one of the greatest medical advances ever made. However, at the end of his life, Pasteur recognized the importance of a healthy terrain—a person's constitution, the internal environment, and the strength to fight off disease—as he famously said on his deathbed, "*Le microbe n'est rien; le terrain est tout*" (translated as "the germ is nothing, the terrain is everything").

Recognizing Vitality Again

The emphasis that many ancient cultures placed on maintaining vitality in life and living a proactively healthy lifestyle made tremendous sense, given the health dangers that existed throughout most of history. Not only did major plagues periodically befall populations and kill off hundreds of thousands, but daily life was also full of risks. Even a simple cold or accidental wound could lead to death. While ancient physicians learned to cure some types of illnesses, most diseases were far beyond their control. As a result, counseling people to stay "vital" was clearly a wise medical philosophy.

Over the past few decades, Western medicine appears to have rediscovered some of the ancient ideas. Despite great technological advances, more and more Western doctors are subscribing to the mind/body relationship and beginning to appreciate the delicate balance between health and illness.

Today, growing numbers of physicians and the public are realizing that good health is a complex phenomenon, and that pharmaceuticals are not cure-alls. More and more medical doctors now recognize that prevention is the single most effective health strategy. We are beginning to understand that good health involves many interactive lifestyle issues, including the very same ones that many ancient cultures emphasized: nutrition, movement, mental attitude, and spiritual beliefs.

Just in the past few decades, several medical doctors such as Andrew Weil and Deepak Chopra have opened our eyes to the wisdom embedded in traditional Chinese and Ayurvedic (Indian) medicine. Their work has enabled us to see that the Western paradigm of medicine is not the only valid one. They have reminded us that these ancient cultures developed effective medical systems based on thousands of years of keen observation of millions of their citizens.

Some of today's best scientific research validates the same knowledge that ancient cultures developed about the human body thousands of years ago. Many American doctors are beginning to accept the notions of qi and prana as our life force or energy force and are increasingly subscribing to some of the fundamental tenets of traditional East Asian medicine, particularly the idea of maintaining vitality in order to live a healthy and long life.

In short, we believe that the ancient concept of vitality can be a valuable metaphor in our life. Even if you don't choose to believe in qi or in the concept of an energy system flowing through pathways in your body, seeking vitality in your life can become one of your most cherished goals. The roots of this wisdom are deep. So, if you have not recently felt a sense of vitality, the rest of this chapter will teach you how to rediscover this healthful state of being.

Regaining Your Vitality

Regaining vitality requires two activities:

- Proper breathing
- Regular walking

We will explain each of these separately and then put them together, so that by the end of this chapter you will learn to do them both at the same time. Walking and breathing in perfect synchrony for thirty minutes to an hour takes concentration. Furthermore, most of us have never truly been taught how to breathe correctly while exercising. Learning these techniques is worth the effort because of the significant health benefits you will gain.

Appreciating the Breath

Unless you are an athlete, a singer, or a dancer, you probably don't think very much about breathing. But breathing properly can be a significant factor in improving our health and adding years to our life. Many ancient cultures took the art of breathing seriously, developing a variety of physical exercises and even spiritual rituals around it. In the East, for example, various deep-breathing techniques were incorporated into many practices of fitness exercise and into the performance arts such as dance. For instance, many martial arts movements in tai chi, kung fu, and qigong require the practitioner to inhale or exhale very slowly in coordination with moving the arms or legs, or to hold the breath for a brief moment to punctuate an intense movement. (By the way, notice that many Chinese exercise techniques have the word *qi* in their name, such as qigong, because these exercises were all developed to harmonize qi, or energy.)

Ancient Indian culture also developed many breathing rituals and practices. Hindu practitioners of yoga also thought that the body contained a life force, called prana, which was absorbed from the air. Yoga practitioners therefore learn the art of pranayama, or controlling the breath, in which they sit in a stationary position, with legs crossed, meditating and breathing in very specific patterns that correlate with their thoughts. It is said that people who are very experienced in yoga can stay healthy with minimal caloric intake because they are able to supplement their nourishment through their practice.

By comparison, Western culture mostly considers breathing strictly on a practical or scientific basis. We think of the breath simply as an exchange of oxygen and carbon dioxide. We respect the biochemical process of breathing, not the mental or emotional connection of the breath to life.

In recent years, however, Western medicine has started to appreciate more complex psychological and physiological issues resulting from improper breathing. For instance, research has taught us that when we are stressed or fearful, our sympathetic nervous system is triggered. This releases the stress hormones that put us in fight-or-flight mode. Our muscles constrict, the heartbeat accelerates, and our chest tightens. We then tend to breathe very shallowly, almost holding our breath as a result of fear or anxiety. This deprives the body and brain of oxygen, clouding our thinking and making us feel uneasy. Such analysis has helped doctors understand how frequent stress can lead to many illnesses such as headaches, back problems, muscle pains, fatigue, and insomnia.

Thus, doctors now teach people who experience a great deal of stress how to engage in slow, deep breathing exercises to relax their bodies and increase their oxygen intake. This helps revert the body to the parasympathetic nervous system, which restores us to a calmer frame of mind.

The contrast between the Eastern and Western approaches to breathing is significant in that it reflects a major difference in how the two cultures understand the essence of being. Throughout the East and now in the West as well, millions of people use precise breathing techniques in association with their fitness exercises, whether the system is yoga or one of the martial arts. In their practices, exercising while coordinating the breath is considered necessary to guard one's health and to preserve one's vitality.

The benefits of breathing properly and efficiently are significant. First, deep breathing keeps the spine and intercostal muscles active and flexible. It also helps increase the level of oxygen entering our lungs. People who breathe deeply feel healthier, more alert, and more energetic. Breathing properly also keeps the lung tissue flexible and moist. Aging tends to make our lungs harden and lose their elasticity, but breathing deeply can improve lung condition and prevent the loss of flexibility. Breathing better also helps the lungs eliminate waste products, preventing them from entering the bloodstream where they can poison cells.

From East Asian medical perspective, reducing waste products helps the kidneys function better and reduces the risks of high blood pressure. A full breath taken from the abdomen also acts as a form of massage for the entire stomach cavity, revitalizing the intestines, stomach, liver, and gallbladder. Finally, breathing deeply helps our appearance and posture, because we tend to hold our spine straighter and not slouch in order to make room in the chest cavity for our lungs.

Proper breathing involves breathing through the nose from the diaphragm (the muscle in the abdomen below the lungs) rather than initiating the breath in the upper chest as most of us do when we breathe in a shallow way. The key is to start your breath from your abdomen, but without straining the diaphragm muscle. As you inhale and naturally tighten your diaphragm, your stomach will go in, and you will automatically expand your rib cage.

This enables your breathing to increase in volume and gives your lungs room to accept all the air coming through your windpipe.

Try the following Vitality Breathing exercise.

1. Sit comfortably on a chair.
2. Drop your arms by your sides and sit up tall so your spine is straight yet comfortable. Let your hands dangle at your sides.
3. As you inhale slowly and deeply through your nose, raise your arms up to your shoulders, as if they are wings and you are about to take flight.
4. Don't breathe too high up in your lungs but rather use your diaphragm to increase the size of your breath.
5. Lower your arms and exhale slowly.

Practicing this type of exercise several times a day will make you more conscious of how shallow and quick your normal breath might be and help you convert it to a deeper, slower breath.

The Vitality Walk

The Vitality Walk presented in this book is derived from two traditions originating in China and in the

Himalayan plateau. The first origin of the Vitality Walk that we teach extends back to the famous physician Hua To in 200 AD, who observed different animals and developed a series of exercises called "animal frolics," each according to a specific walking style. One of Hua To's precepts was that correct breathing must accompany physical movement to maximize its effectiveness.

The second origin of the Vitality Walk that we teach comes from a walking style developed by caravanning nomads in the mountainous regions of Hunza Valley at the base of the Himalayas. Living and traveling at high altitudes above six thousand feet, these nomads often walk up to twenty miles a day, traveling from village to village to sell their goods. To adapt to the harsh conditions, the nomads created a synchronized walking/breathing pattern that the French researcher Edouard Stiegler characterized as providing "suroxygenation," meaning a higher level of oxygen to the blood.[1] Stiegler stated that the physical, mental, and spiritual benefits of this type of breathing and walking are enormous, helping people achieve significantly increased vitality, better sleep, and stronger resistance to disease.

The Vitality Walk does not require that you walk as fast as the supercharged methods that some

American walking advocates teach (e.g., power walking, aerobic walking, or Japanese walking). You do not need to pump or flail your arms, or vigorously spring off your toes as you take each step, as such high-powered methods require.

The Vitality Walk only needs to be done at a steady, healthy walking pace. However, this doesn't mean that you are slowly strolling. A too-slow pace obviously won't yield real benefits. But you do not need to walk exaggeratedly fast or even approach running speed (five miles per hour).

Furthermore, the Vitality Walk does not ask you to be concerned with any statistical measures, such as your heart rate or caloric burn rate. Don't think about your speed or the distance you cover. You don't need to jog. Briskly walking one mile in fifteen minutes burns about the same number of calories as jogging an equal distance in eight minutes. However, slowly increasing your walking speed is a valuable goal, as it does produce more dramatic conditioning effects.

Once again, the most important goal is to rejuvenate your inner vitality, which cannot be measured, only felt. For this reason, the pace, duration, and level of difficulty of your walk is entirely dependent on you. You do not need to take your pulse, count your heartbeat, or calculate a target heart rate for your age and weight.

Instead, the goal of a Vitality Walk is to allow your mind/body to become aware of your inner energy so you can circulate it throughout your body and revitalize yourself. Simply walk and pay attention to the sensation of energy emanating from inside you for whatever amount of time you are comfortable walking.

While this idea of feeling your vitality—your qi—may sound strange to you, especially if you are not familiar with East Asian medicine, it is not very different than feeling the physical sensations your body gives you when you are exhausted after a hard day at work or revved up before a big event. We all become aware of such feelings because our bodies clearly communicate them to us. We intuitively sense it when we are tired, excited, or charged up. The same goes for feeling your vitality; you can tell when you have it—and when you don't.

As you go on your Vitality Walks, concentrate on the breathing patterns you will learn in this chapter because they will help clear your mind and focus on feeling what your body communicates to you. With experience, you will increasingly feel your muscles and limbs moving, your blood flowing, the cells in your lungs breathing, and a core of energy pulsing through you. The more Vitality Walks you take, the more in touch you will become with this inner core of energy—and the more of this energy you will emanate.

Preparing for the Vitality Walk

To prepare for a Vitality Walk, follow these general instructions and watch the video provided here.

1. Warm up first by breathing deeply as explained in the vitality breathing exercise on page 39. This short warm-up helps you clear your mind and begin focusing on your breath.
2. Warm up your knee joints. Bend your knees gently so that your palms are resting on your knees and massage the knees and surrounding tissue with your hands in a circular motion, both clockwise and counterclockwise for a minute or more.

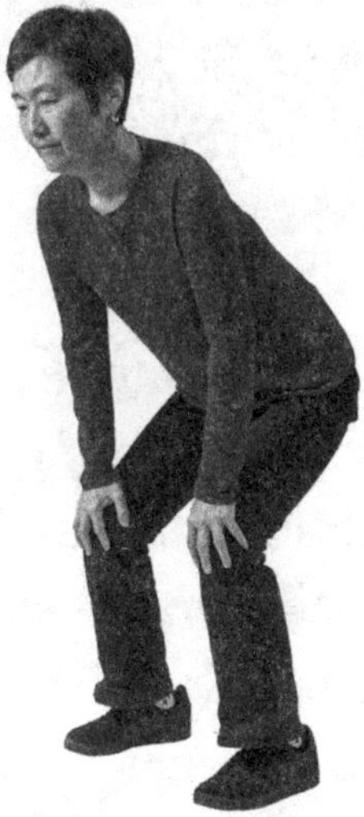

3. Raise and lower your arms a few times to limber your upper body. Then flex your

knees and point your toes to stretch out your leg muscles.

Get ready to walk. If you can, go outside to do the walk. Of course, it is easier and more enjoyable to walk when the weather is good and the sun is shining, but many people throughout the world exercise even in the rain and the cold of winter. If the weather in your area is especially cold or rainy, consult the appendix for clothing options. Here are the guidelines for how you set up your body to perform this walk:

Hand Position

When you walk, position your arms comfortably at your sides. Close your hands in loose fists but tuck your thumbs gently inside. In the Yogic tradition, this hand position is called the Adi Mudra. This mudra promotes well-being and concentration and connects to the lung region to help improve breathing and circulation and energizes your movement. (Different hand positions or mudras in the Yogic tradition are said to create an energy, or prana, circuit. Think of the circle position made, using the first finger touching the thumb when people meditate and say the mantra "om.")

Hand Position for Vitality Walk

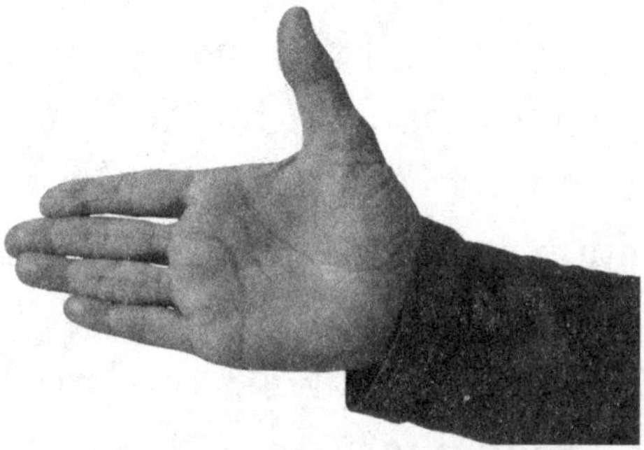

Begin with your hand in an open position.

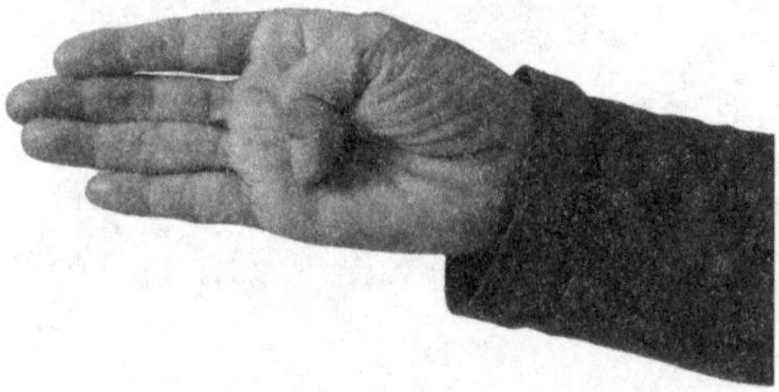

Gently tuck your thumb into your palm.

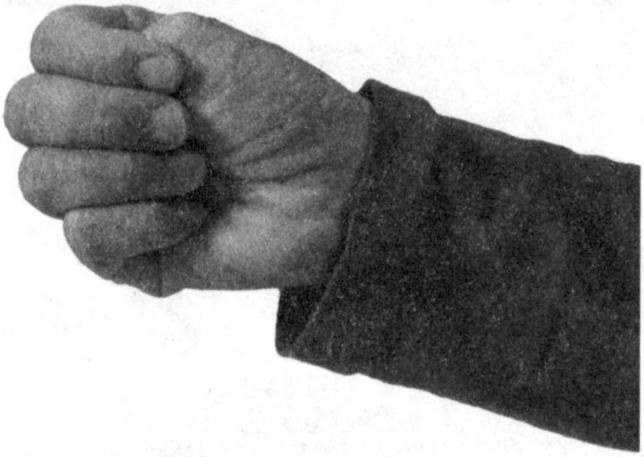

Now close your hand loosely.

Tongue

Curl your tongue slightly so that the tip touches the roof of your mouth, as if you were forming the letter "l." Keeping your tongue in this position helps you secrete saliva as you walk, reducing your thirst. This tongue position will feel awkward at first, but with time you will be able to hold it comfortably. If it feels very uncomfortable, simply let your tongue sit normally in your mouth for now, until you feel ready to try it again.

Feet

As you walk, place one foot in front of the other, placing your heel down first and rolling your foot to the toe. Don't try to walk a fine line as if you were on a tightrope or balance beam. That type of foot pattern is very unnatural. Just place one foot in front of the other, with each foot landing a few inches off an imaginary center line that you are following.

Stance

As you walk, stand up fairly straight; don't round your back or shoulders because that slows you down. Similarly, don't intentionally lean forward in an effort to walk faster. These positions strain the back muscles. Also, keep your head up and focus your eyes about ten to fifteen feet in front of you. Don't tilt your head down; this also strains the back and neck muscles. The breathing patterns you will learn here will help with your body positioning.

Breathing

The Vitality Walk generally has you inhale and exhale through your nose, not through your mouth. Inhaling through your mouth puts dry air into your lungs, which tends to make breathing difficult. Some of the breathing patterns you will learn below ask that you not simply inhale through your nose, but rather that you vigorously sniff the air through your nostrils. Sniffing the air actually gives better oxygenation and helps with your concentration. Vigorous sniffing may feel uncomfortable at first, especially if you have clogged nasal passages or a cold. Vigorous sniffing will also cause you to feel like you have a runny nose, so bring some tissues with you. Eventually, you will see that sniffing in air actually increases your intake and opens up your nasal passages.

Two Levels of the Vitality Walk

We have created two levels of the Vitality Walk. We recommend you try each one and see which one is best for you. There is a video demonstrating each level of the walk. Keep in mind that there is no time allotment, at least initially. You can do this walking style for as long as you enjoy the experience, without regard to your heart rate or pulse. If you walk for only five to ten minutes when you are first starting out, that's fine. You can then build up to longer walks of twenty to thirty minutes or longer as you improve your conditioning and gain increasing ability to feel your inner vitality.

The Basic Vitality Walk

This level is intended for everyone, without regard to age, ability, or physical health. This is an introductory walk in which you simply learn to walk and breathe at the same time.

The basic Vitality Walk is a five-step cycle. As you walk, you sniff in as you take each of the first two steps, then exhale by sniffing out on the third step, then hold an empty lung position on the fourth and fifth steps. A summary of this walk is as follows:

- First step: sniff in
- Second step: sniff in again
- Third step: exhale by sniffing out
- Fourth and fifth steps: neutral breath position (your lungs are empty, and you are breathing neither in nor out)

Once you begin doing this walk, you will see that the first sniff fills your lungs about halfway, and the second sniff finishes filling them. You will then feel the need to exhale very naturally on the third step. This exhale should be large enough to decompress your chest and lungs in a natural manner. You will feel almost like you are blowing your nose vigorously with both nostrils.

Note: if your nostrils are clogged, you may want to blow your nose before you start on your walk to clear them out. As you proceed, you will find that your nostrils will open more, and you may need to blow your nose again. Over time, this walk will help you achieve better breathing and clearer nasal passages, unless you have an obstruction such as polyps or a deviated septum.

The fourth and fifth steps are a momentary hiatus in breathing to complete the cycle. Do not exhale or inhale any air. These steps are intended to give your lungs a rest and a break in the pattern. This is not the same as holding your breath, which is usually done after having inhaled. In this case, you are in "neutral breath," not breathing in or out while the lungs are empty from the preceding exhalation.

One unusual aspect of this walk is that the two sniffs followed by the exhale end up making a rhythmic marching sound that helps to drive you forward. You will feel and hear the cadence as you walk. This first level of the Vitality Walk will invigorate you enormously if you do it for as little as five minutes or one-quarter of a mile. You may practice as long as you are comfortable.

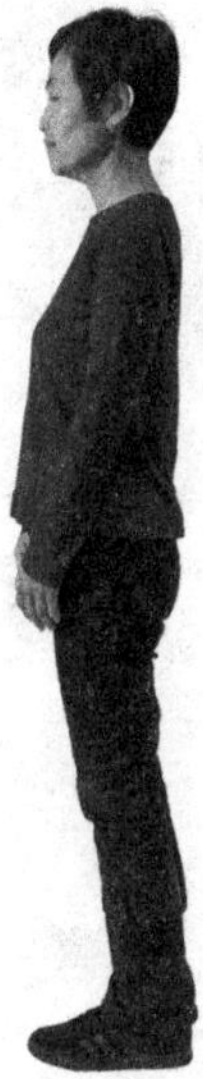

This is your starting position for the Vitality Walk. Notice the alignment of the spine. You are not slouched forward; your spine is erect and you have a feeling of elongation as if pulled from the top of your head.

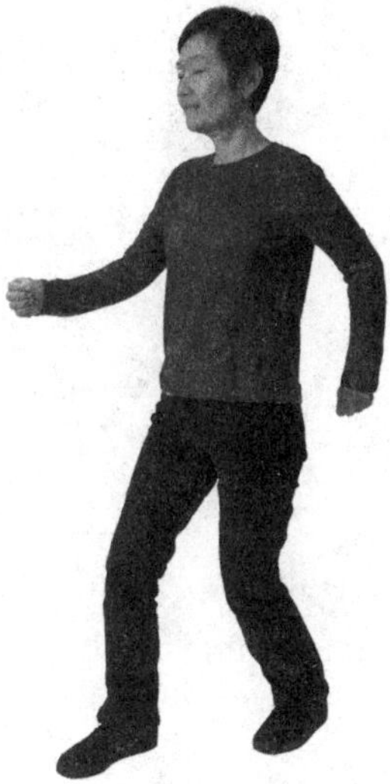

You step forward with your right (or left) foot, and sniff in as you might if you were inhaling an aroma of a wonderful flower.

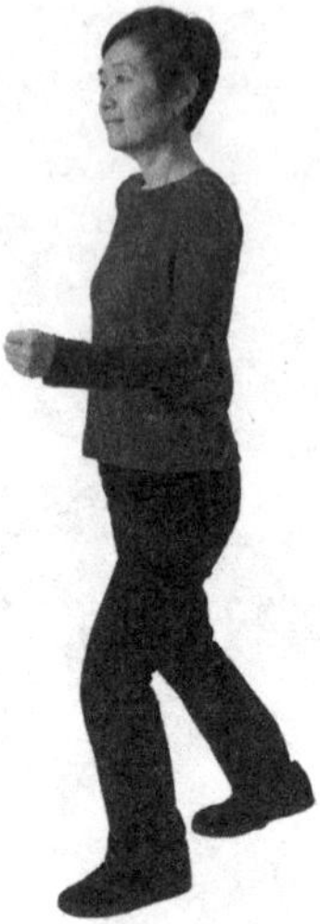

Next, step forward with your opposite foot and sniff in again.

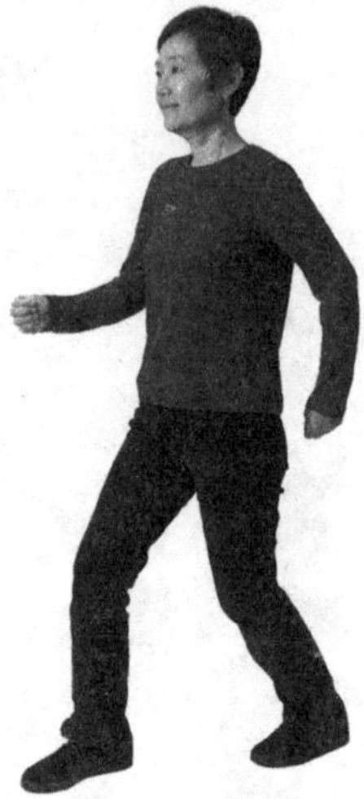

As you step again, you sniff out to clear your lungs completely. There is some vigor in this exhalation.

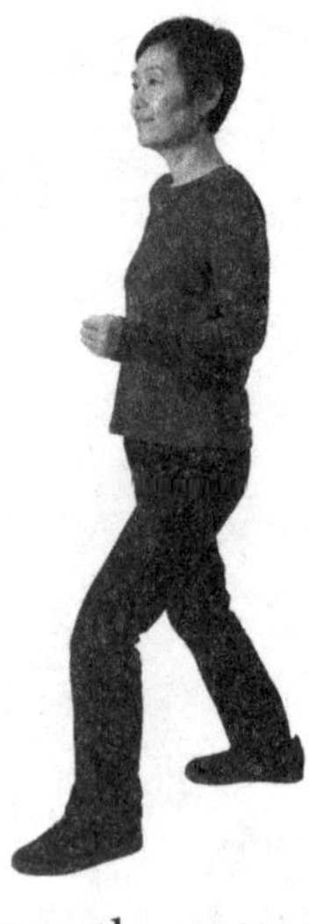

Continue the pattern as you proceed with the Vitality Walk.

The Moderate Vitality Walk

This level of the Vitality Walk is closest to the highest region of the Himalayan plateau. It differs from the basic Vitality Walk in the breathing pattern it uses, which makes the pace slightly quicker. This is an eight-step walk, and it does not use sniffing, but rather continuous inhaling/exhaling through your nose.

For the first three steps, you inhale the entire time through your nose to fill your lungs. On the fourth step, you are in neutral breath position, breathing neither in nor out. On the next three steps, you exhale slowly. On the final step, you are in neutral breath again. The pattern for this walk is:

- First step: start inhaling
- Second and third step: continue inhaling
- Fourth step: neutral breath position
- Fifth step: start exhaling
- Sixth and seventh step: continue exhaling
- Eighth step: neutral breath position

The value of this level of the Vitality Walk is that it oxygenates your system more completely and stimulates your circulation more than the basic Vitality Walk. This is because you breathe in over three steps rather than two, thus filling your lungs even more deeply. The neutral position at the third inhale and exhale finish points also gives your lungs and heart a momentary rest, so they are not taxed too much.

WEEK 3
The Mindfulness Walk for Inner Peace

There is a path from your mind to your heart—walk it with your feet.

—Rumi

In this chapter, we will explore the Mindfulness Walk. This walk is aimed at developing a greater sense of inner peace by helping you focus on psychological and spiritual rebalancing. It is an awareness walk that promotes equanimity and reduces the damaging effects of stress hormones on the body. Learning this walk will help you be in the moment, quiet the mind, match your breathing to your steps, and feel joy as you walk. The Mindfulness Walk includes specific positions of the hands that aid in achieving a meditative state of mind. It can be its own style of walking for your entire daily walk, or it can be a segment of your traditional daily walk.

The Mindfulness Walk can be traced to the Buddhist tradition, which emphasizes meditation and the cultivation of the mind toward peace and liberation. Mindfulness, however, is not a religious concept. It is a state of being that allows you to be fully awake and to be present with your experiences.

What Is Mindfulness?

Mindfulness is an inner experience of being closely in touch with your awareness of the present moment. It is letting go of your thinking about the past or the future. You observe only what is in front of you, accepting whatever the situation is, without judgment. Being mindful is to be aware of feelings such as anxiety, recrimination, guilt, worry, or shame, without adding a layer of judgment about these feelings. When you are mindful, you become aware of the constant self-talk that dominates our usual waking hours.

The popularization of mindfulness in Western culture began in the late 1970s with Jon Kabat-Zinn, a molecular biologist, who was a student of Korean Buddhism, Vipassana meditation, and yoga. He had a vision of bringing mindfulness into mainstream medical care, and in 1979, he began teaching mindfulness practices to patients with chronic pain at the University of Massachusetts Medical School in Worcester. As a scientist, he understood the importance of research, and he conducted studies where he demonstrated that people who were trying to avoid pain typically worsened the pain rather than relieving it. His program, Mindfulness-Based Stress Reduction (MBSR), taught patients to observe the pain, to be present with it, and to release their story about the pain. This proved to be a more successful approach. The MBSR classes taught patients that what we resist persists and that the act of paying attention to the breath when meditating and focusing on the feet when walking had the result of reducing pain. The use of mindfulness has since expanded into numerous other medical areas and therapies.

Mindfulness is an inner experience without performance goals. The goal of mindfulness is simply *to be*.

The Benefits of the Mindfulness Walk

When you make the Mindfulness Walk a part of your walking regimen, you are likely to experience many of the following benefits:

Stress Reduction

We often juggle a lot of responsibilities and, as a result, become stressed. As we discussed earlier, stress has been shown to be a factor in numerous health problems, including heart disease, gastrointestinal problems, headaches, and back pain. One of the best ways to release stress is through a calming practice, such as Mindfulness Walking. This style of walking allows both mental and muscle tension to be released so that you can relax. Mental tension is reduced as our thoughts slow down and then are quieted. A relaxing effect spreads across your entire physical body as you release the concerns of your daily life that cause tension in your neck and shoulders.

Centering of the Mind and Soul

Mindfulness helps us to notice the streams of our self-talk, which is often negative and self-critical. When you develop your awareness, you can begin to change and redirect your mind. You can become more grounded in your positive beingness, feeding both the mind and the soul. In addition, when you are feeling more centered, solutions to problems may come more easily. You are less likely to be thrown off-balance by a change of plans or an unforeseen obstacle.

Reduced Depression

Many experiments have been conducted to learn if mindfulness training can contribute to alleviating depression. One study showed that mindfulness can reduce the prevalence of depressive rumination, in which the person is unable to control continuously thinking negative thoughts. In that study, fifty out of eighty participants learned mindfulness practices to regulate their attention and present-moment awareness as a treatment for depression; the other thirty participants were given standard psychological treatment for depression. Magnetic resonance imaging (MRI) of the participants' brains showed that those who learned mindfulness had less connectivity in a neural network associated with depressive rumination compared to those receiving standard care. The study found that practicing present-moment awareness led to reduction in overly negative thinking causing depression.[1]

Heightened Awareness and Appreciation for Life

At the heart of the Mindfulness Walk is the potential to experience life at a very high level. As you train the mind, you can become less preoccupied by your daily worries, and you can have a more direct experience of being present to life. Released from the shadow of anxiety and worry, you can delight in the variety and wonder of the surrounding world. A sense of joy begins to seep into your consciousness.

Bodily Regeneration and Replenishment

Physiological activity is a necessary part of well-being. Our bodies must replenish themselves to operate at an optimal level. Regeneration is a complex activity involving the production and release of energy, the processing of food, the transformation of old cells into new ones, the elimination of waste by-products, and other functions. Nutrition and oxygen play important roles in the regeneration process. Mindfulness Walking and other meditation practices allow our central nervous system to relax. As a result, blood circulation and breathing are enhanced. This promotes regeneration and helps us feel more alert and alive.

Direct Physical Benefits

Along with the benefits of the meditative aspects of the Mindfulness Walk, there are also some general physical gains from the simple act of walking. Walking is a great means of achieving overall conditioning, and it is particularly good for strengthening the lower body. It can lower your risk of death from several common conditions, including stroke and high blood pressure. Walking strengthens bones and heart muscle, which improves their performance. It slows aging and the general decline of the body. For those with type 2 diabetes, walking can decrease the need for insulin. Walking also increases energy and stamina.

Preparing to Do the Mindfulness Walk

The Mindfulness Walk is often described as a moving meditation. Here are some recommendations that will help you prepare to do this walk.

Be in the Moment

Slow down and be present in your immediate experience. There is no need to hurry or to arrive anywhere in particular. What's most important is that your mind is aware that you are on a walk. Allow yourself to experience the delight of your movement. Your connection to your own true experience will be increasingly direct.

Find Ways to Quiet Your Mind

It is normal and natural for your brain to be constantly absorbing information from your senses and processing it in the form of thoughts, feelings, and memories. Rather than trying to turn off your mind, halting all such brain functions, the invitation is to simply allow the thoughts to come and go.

There are many methods to work with your thoughts to slow them down. One approach that works well when you begin practicing the Mindfulness Walk is to count the number of steps you take with each breath. Counting steps allows you to focus on your breathing, not your thoughts, while maintaining movement.

Here's how counting the steps works: Slow your walking down to the same pace as your breathing. Walk in this style for several minutes. Next, begin to take note of the number of steps you take as you inhale and exhale. Concentrating on the steps taken will calm your mind and help you focus on the present moment, not your thoughts.

Breathe Naturally

Take natural but deep breaths. Breathe into your abdomen. Observe your breath and allow it to assist in relaxing your body. If it feels natural, allow your inhalation to last longer than your exhalation. If there is a partial step during each breath, then adjust your pace or breathing so that you end up with a

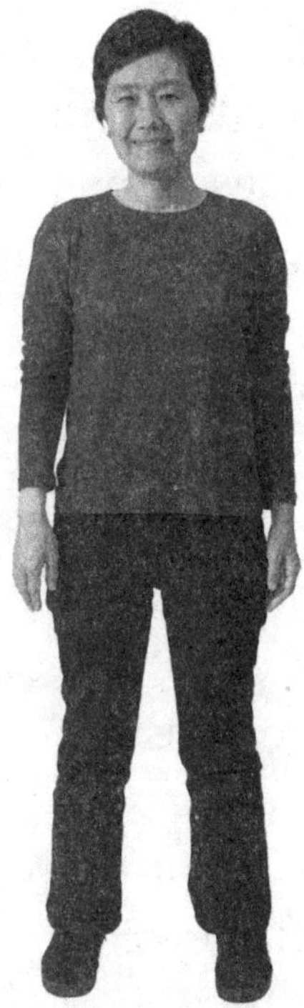

whole number. You can also vary your pace in different segments of your walk. Once you have been doing the walking practice for a while, you might extend the exhalation to equal the inhalation by adding an extra step for that section of your breath. Try this for just five breaths or so once in a while during your walk.

Another method is to simply count the breaths from one to ten. Inhalations and exhalations can be included as one count or counted separately. Once you reach ten, start counting again. If you lose track (which can be easy to do), simply begin anew at one.

An alternative to counting steps is to silently repeat a short phrase of aspiration that matches your pace, such as "May I step with joy," "May I be healthy and strong," "May I move with grace and ease," or "May I be grounded." Choose words and a beat that feel right for you.

All these methods are helpful in creating an inner silence and transporting you out of your head and into experiencing the world around you.

Smile as You Move

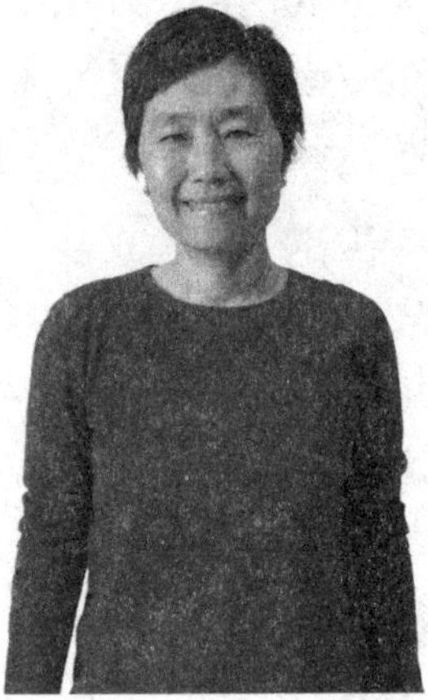

Walking with a gentle inner or outer smile will lighten your spirit. The smile is also another point of attention that can quiet your mind. As you let go of your daily concerns, your body will relax more and more. Allow yourself to be comfortable. Visualize yourself walking with confidence

Step into Joy

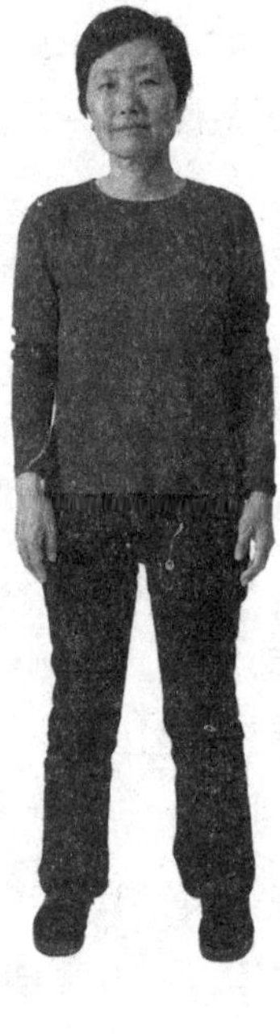

If possible, try to practice the Mindfulness Walk outdoors to connect with nature and enhance your experience. Attune yourself to the beauty of the natural environment that surrounds you. Notice all of its diversity in the colors, smells, and sounds. If you begin your walk feeling burdened with worry, imagine a pleasant breeze flowing over you and taking your worries away as it drifts past. Feel joy taking up the space that worry left behind. Allow each step to express this joy. Moving with joy during your walk will help you live in joy during your day-to-day life.

Let Worries Go

When worried thoughts remain with you, you may want to begin walking with determination. Breathe comfortably and know that you are entitled to experience inner peace. Recognize your struggle, feel compassion for yourself, and understand that things are just as they are.

Become the Movement

In mindfulness, there is also the idea of "non-doing." What this means is that whatever activity you are involved in, you become. When on a Mindfulness Walk, you become one with the walk. A sense of self dissolves so that you are harmoniously and totally involved in the movement.

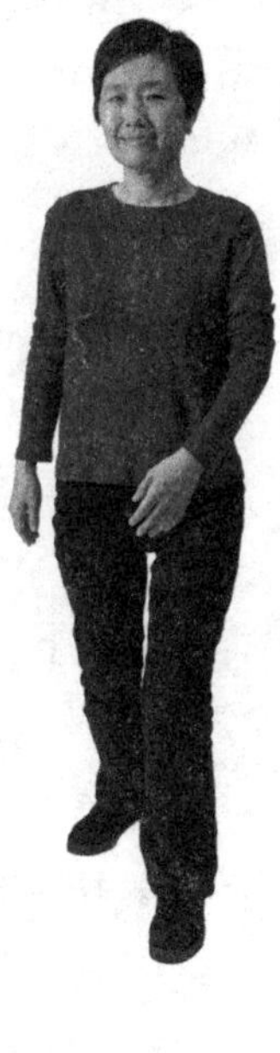

How to Do the Mindfulness Walk

If possible, choose a peaceful, quiet outdoor location for your walk. Areas near a lake or the ocean and paths through parks and forests are ideal. You want a fairly flat terrain so that you can concentrate on the meditative aspect of your walk. If you are unable to walk in a natural environment, be sure your location will provide a pleasant atmosphere.

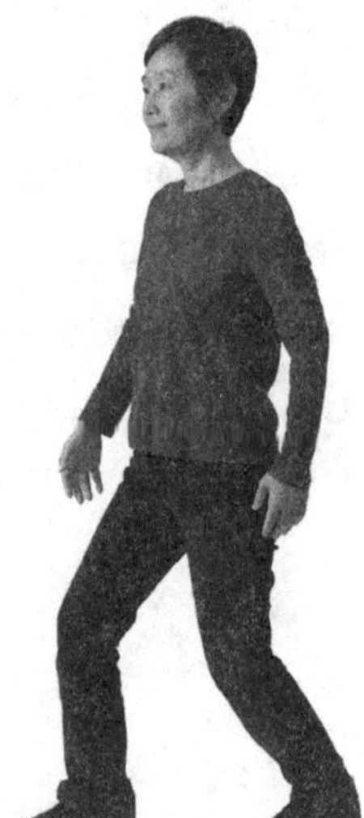

1. Stand still for a few moments and breathe calmly. Begin to focus on the present moment and quiet your thoughts to help yourself get ready to enter a state of mindfulness. Take some slow, deep breaths and look skyward. This will help you calm your thoughts.
2. Place your hands in what is called the "half a prayer" position. Your dominant hand

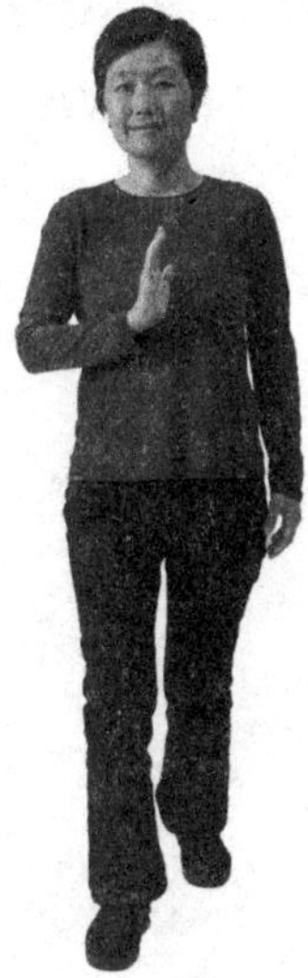

(the hand you use most of the time, such as when writing) is placed upright at your chest, as though that hand was praying alone, while the other hand hangs relaxed at your side.

3. Now begin walking at a slow pace, breathing comfortably and deeply into your abdomen. Let go of any tension in the body if you are able. Be aware of the landing of your feet. Feel each heel make contact with the ground (or floor) as well as the roll-out as you land on the balls of your feet. As each foot lands, visualize energy coming into the sole of your foot from the earth. The landing of your foot massages what is known as the Kidney 1 (Chinese: Yong Quan-Gushing Spring) acupuncture point on the sole of the foot. In traditional Chinese medicine, the kidney is important in maintaining the body's energy.
4. Continue walking in a slow, peaceful, and joyful manner. Smile gently. Sink deeper into your inner essence.

5. Begin to notice the details of the natural world around you. Be aware of all your senses. Start with your sense of sight, taking in the colors and variety of the visual world around you. Then move to your sense of smell; can you detect the scent of the air? Do you smell flowers, trees, freshly mown grass, or damp earth? How about sounds? Are there birds warbling, bees buzzing, water gurgling, or gentle breezes whispering to you? Take all of this in as if you had never experienced it before. Allow your awareness to increase as you relax more and more.
6. Keep strolling slowly for the duration of your walk. If you would like, add the counting practice or repeat the aspirational phrases practice described above. Stay in the moment and enjoy each step invigorated with life.

* * *

This is similar to the basic mindfulness walk, but it uses an alternative hand position.

1. Stand still for a few moments and breathe calmly. Focus on the present moment and quiet your thoughts. Take some slow, deep breaths and look skyward. This will help you calm your thoughts.
2. Place your hands in the "cosmic mudra" (a.k.a. Dhyana) position, where your dominant hand is held at your lower abdomen, palm up. In the palm of the dominant hand lies the other hand, also palm up. Put your thumbs together, touching lightly and forming an oval.

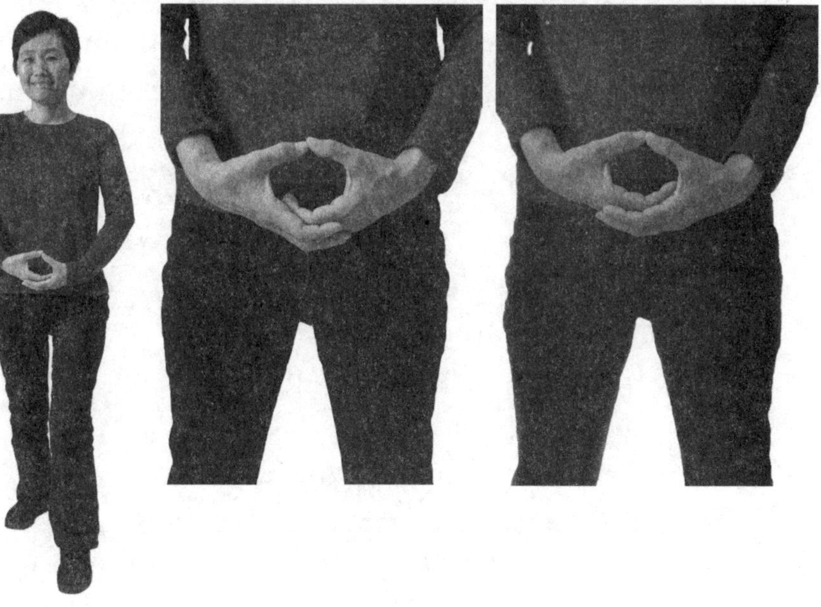

3. Begin walking at a slow pace, just as with the prior Mindfulness Walk. Breathe comfortably and deeply into your abdomen. Let go of any tension in the body.
4. Continue walking in a slow, peaceful, and joyful manner. Smile gently. Sink deeper into your inner essence.

Start with short sessions of the Mindfulness Walk that last only about ten minutes. Gradually, if you wish, you can increase the lengths of walks to as much as an hour. With regular practice, you will be amazed at how much you can quiet your mind as your senses open up to the environment around you. You will also begin to notice moments of heightened awareness even when you are not walking.

Other Ways to Practice Mindfulness

The mindful awareness and consciousness you develop from this walk can be applied to any activity you do—eating, drinking tea, viewing an art exhibit, playing a sport, or listening to music. You can create that same sense of inner stillness and being open to the moment, without feeling distracted by your thoughts, feelings, or memories of the past or future. Simply enjoy the activity as it comes to you without filters. Just be there and experience it. Become more and more alive. As a dear friend, the author Bernard Gunther, described it, "Let go of all content, and you will be totally content."

The more you practice mindfulness in other activities of your life, the more skillful you may also become during your Mindfulness Walks. In this way, the benefits of mindfulness may multiply, helping you become calmer, more balanced, healthier, and free.

Week 4
The Immune Power Walk to Optimize Health

Walking is a person's best medicine.
—Hippocrates

For five thousand years, people in Asia have turned to qigong (pronounced chi-gong), a combination of movement and breathing to bolster their health and help ward off illness. Shamanic dances in early tribal rituals and celebrations may have been an ancient forerunner to qigong. Performing the dances was seen as a way to relieve the aches and pains of arthritis and to maintain a strong body. Over time, specific moves were created to be used as treatments for particular illnesses and imbalances. Such qigong-type medical practices predate acupuncture. *The Yellow Emperor's*

Classic of Internal Medicine, written in the third century BCE, describes exercise and breathing techniques that could help maintain wellness and assist in self-healing.

For much of its history, qigong was only available to the elite. Over the centuries, physicians associated with various dynasties shared their knowledge of qigong-like practices with royalty and the members of the court to support health and fight illness. Specific body movements were taught along with particular breathing patterns.

These techniques have evolved into what is known today as the medical version of qigong. Currently, there is a resurgence of interest throughout the world in this approach to treating various medical conditions. The techniques of qigong are being used both by people who want to continue to live in good health and by those whose health is challenged by disease or illness.

In this chapter, we will introduce two qigong walks that are beneficial as moderate exercise for individuals seeking to improve general health and to develop flexibility. Also, they are currently used to treat many chronic conditions caused by a weakened immune system, in particular, as part of the treatment for some types of cancer.

The Story of Guo Lin Medical Qigong

The two walks we are teaching you are both derived from a Chinese artist named Guo Lin, born in 1909. In the 1940s, her life took an unforeseen turn when she was diagnosed with uterine cancer, and she underwent a hysterectomy. Her cancer returned after ten years, having metastasized into her bladder. With a strong desire to live, Guo Lin sought a variety of solutions based on both Eastern and Western medicine. She underwent six surgeries, but nothing halted the cancer growth. She was finally told that she had just six months to live.

Searching for answers, Guo Lin began using the qigong practices that her grandfather had taught her as a child. She also studied both traditional Chinese medicine (TCM) and Western medicine and began to apply what she had learned from them to her qigong walks. She experimented with various movements and breathing techniques, ultimately creating her own unique form of qigong movements. Within six months, her cancer went into remission. Guo Lin felt that it was the qigong that had enabled her to live when her primary doctors and oncologists thought she would not survive.

Inspired, Guo Lin went on to teach her version of qigong to many others over the following twenty years. She passed away from other causes on December 14, 1984, but her namesake organization, the Guo Lin Research Society, estimates that over one million cancer patients practice her form of medical qigong every day. Groups of people with cancer meet in parks throughout China to work out together. The sounds they make while practicing the movements fill the air with a chorus of "Chee chee hoo," meaning "inhale, inhale, exhale."

Guo Lin qigong is often recommended by oncologists in China in addition to conventional cancer treatments. The Guo Lin Research Society reports that a consistent and diligent practice of qigong lessens the side effects of chemotherapy, increases appetite, and creates a feeling of well-being in patients.

Since Guo Lin, the medical practice of qigong has continued to spread throughout the world. Numerous international conferences have been held for researchers and practitioners, including at the University of California, Berkeley, and at Harvard. Contemporary research supports the benefits of qigong for immune support.

Health Benefits of Qigong

The health benefits of a qigong walking practice stem from three foundational principles:

- When doing one of the Immune Power Walks, you exercise the entire body, delivering healthful benefits to various organs and bodily systems, including the immune system.
- The movements and breathing patterns are designed to strengthen your qi energy, giving you an internal boost of vitality.
- Finally, qigong, particularly Guo Lin qigong, is often performed as a group activity that provides emotional and social support for a sense of well-being.

Let's look in detail at how the medical benefits of qigong flow from these three principles.

General Healthful Benefits to the Entire Body

Research reports that qigong positively affects the brain, heart, kidney, and immune system, providing benefits to patients with diabetes, chronic obstructive pulmonary disease, hypertension, stroke, cervical spondylosis, lumbar disc herniation, insomnia, knee osteoarthritis, low back pain, osteoporosis, coronary heart disease, breast cancer, periarthritis of shoulder, depression, and metabolic syndrome.[1] Specifically, the movements and breathing patterns of qigong help regulate the sympathetic and parasympathetic nervous system. When the nervous system is calmed, your heartbeat is moderated, blood pressure lowers, respiration deepens, and digestive processes improve. In this way, your entire body benefits from the state of tranquility brought about by the practice.

Another healing aspect of qigong is that it releases tension held in the muscles and other body tissues. Chronic contraction of tissues impedes the movement of blood, lymph fluid, and immune substances throughout the body. Cellular metabolism is also diminished when the body is tense. Qigong's gentle movements massage the tissues, allowing better functioning of these various processes.

There's also no doubt that regular walking contributes to longevity. In one Finnish study held over a period of nineteen years, even occasional walking—about six half-hour walks per month—led to 30 percent less likelihood of death compared to nonactivity.[2]

Supporting Immunity

Qigong is often used as an adjunct treatment for diseases, including cancer, in combination with traditional medical approaches. New research provides evidence that qigong can have a positive impact on supporting the immune system. Research indicates that exercise may play a role in preventing cancer. Several studies have verified that physically active people are less likely to get certain types of cancer.[3] In fact, the American Cancer Society recommends exercise as one way to reduce the risk of cancer. Some ill people are unable to do strenuous exercise, and more and more studies indicate that pushing hard may not be necessary to help fight disease. In some cases, strenuous exercise—such as running a marathon—has shown to decrease immune functioning, at least initially. As a result, many patients turn to the soft, flowing movements of qigong. There are numerous reports from patients who say that the Guo Lin qigong practices have helped to facilitate their recovery from cancer and other chronic illnesses.

1. Various studies have also documented that certain types of exercise support the immune system by promoting the production of cancer-fighting white blood cells called *lymphocytes*. Levels of *lymphokines*, chemicals that stimulate lymphocyte activity, have also been shown to regulate immunity.

Qigong also increases the production of cyclic adenosine monophosphate (CAMP), a chemical that transforms cancer cells into normal cells. The body's ability to rid itself of harmful bacteria and viruses is also given support.

2. Another study using nineteen participants who learned to practice qigong for fourteen weeks showed that the exercise lowered the stress-hormone cortisol levels, which helps to increase the production of cytokine-secreting cells that help support immunity. Other studies have shown that qigong improves the production of T cells and natural killer (NK) cells.[4]
3. It is well known that your emotional state affects the physiological functions of your body. In researching the emotional history of cancer patients, it was observed that many of them had previously survived trauma prior to the cancer diagnosis, and when the cancer occurred, they were prone to depression, anxiety, worries, and pessimism. It was concluded therefore that if the emotional state of a cancer patient were to change to a more positive one, it may help slow the

cancer growth. A strong belief in being able to manage cancer through a regular practice of qigong, along with remaining calm, relaxed and unaffected by the environment, can help survival. As stated above, studies have shown that qigong helps lower cortisol production, which aids in reducing a well-known consequence of cancer treatment, cancer-related fatigue (CRF) resulting from sleep disorders, depression, stress, and anxiety in cancer survivors. Exercise also increases the output of endorphins, the body's "feel-good" natural biochemicals, which are thought to play a role in fighting cancer.

Nurturing Qi Energy

Many ancient traditions believe there is a "life force" energy that fuels us. As we cited before, traditional Chinese medicine (TCM) calls it *qi* while Ayurvedic medicine in India calls it *prana*, the Sanskrit word for breath. According to Chinese medicine tradition, the life force energy travels through the body along a system of channels called meridians. The flow of *qi* circulates on a twenty-four-hour schedule and varies depending on seasonal cycles. In this system of medicine, disease is viewed as the result of blockages that prevent the flow of qi to the organs of the body.

In traditional Chinese medicine, the central storage place for qi is an area known as the *Dan Tian,* located about four finger widths below the navel. This area is one of the more important of the seven hundred energy points that have been identified and used in acupuncture, acupressure, and qigong. The movements and breathing patterns of qigong were devised in part to stimulate the circulation of energy and air throughout the body and to promote the process of self-healing.

Building qi is often compared to putting money in a savings account. The more energy you accumulate, the stronger and healthier you will feel. When starting a qigong practice, it is useful to try to sense this flow of energy in your body. Some people are able to pick up on this energy very quickly, whereas others never do. If you're having difficulty, picture in your mind the flow of energy throughout your body and see if you can learn to sense the shifts in it. Don't worry if you can never actually detect it. Just trust the process.

Group Support to Fight Disease

Guo Lin qigong is performed as a group activity, which gives participants an opportunity to share their experiences with others who are dealing with similar challenges. This emotional support is thought to be a factor in the recovery process. Also, the informal exchange of information lessens the stress experienced by those gathered. Seeing others survive and even thrive despite their cancer diagnosis gives people hope. (Note: it is not necessary to practice qigong in a group setting in order to receive its benefits.)

In a research proposal to examine the role of qigong on cancer-related fatigue, published in the May 2024 issue of the medical journal *Integrative Cancer Therapies*, the researchers synthesized the positive effects of qigong in this way:

> All forms of Qigong involve the recognition and cultivation of Qi to promote a balanced Qi and smooth flow of Qi in the body to enhance physical, psychological, and spiritual health through mind-body integration of specific movements, breathing techniques, and meditation. Mind-body integration of Qigong is also believed to promote health through the activation of neurohormonal pathways and other physiological mechanisms. Qigong offers several potential advantages

to supplement modern medical therapy as it emphasizes a holistic approach with minimal adverse effects when practiced correctly after proper guidance. It is also known to improve neuropsychiatric conditions without the side effects that can occur with pharmaceutical drugs. More importantly, it promotes self-empowerment as it empowers individuals to take an active role in their health. Lastly, Qigong is a cost-effective supplement to certain medical treatments, because once learned, it can be practiced regularly to promote a healthy lifestyle without the need to incur additional expenses.[5]

Importance of the Breath in Qigong

Breathing exercises, either combined with physical movements or on their own, have been practiced since ancient times in many cultures. Today, breathwork—learning how to intentionally modify your breathing patterns—continues to be a subject of extensive medical research in the treatment of sleep disorders, chronic disease, anxiety, depression, and much more.

Breathing is an essential aspect of all qigong practices, including the two Immune Power Walks you will learn in this chapter. Its very name comes from two root words, "qi" and "gong" which can be translated as "breath practice."

To warm up for the two Immune Power Walks, you will learn a deep abdominal breathing pattern to relax any tension you are holding in your body as you prepare for movement. Then the two actual walks use a special breathing pattern similar to the one for the Vitality Walk we previously covered in chapter 2. This pattern involves inhaling twice through the nose for every breath you release. This maximizes the amount of oxygen you take into your body so that your qi, your life force energy, will be nourished by the air you bring in.

Before we begin exploring the qigong walks, it helps to examine the way you breathe in your everyday life. Are you breathing deeply enough? Remember, it's important to engage your diaphragm (the muscles in the abdomen below the lungs) when breathing, rather than just using your upper chest.

One simple way to see whether you are fully using your diaphragm when you breathe is to simply place one hand beneath your navel and the other on your chest. Do both your chest and abdomen rise just slightly when you inhale? If so, your breathing

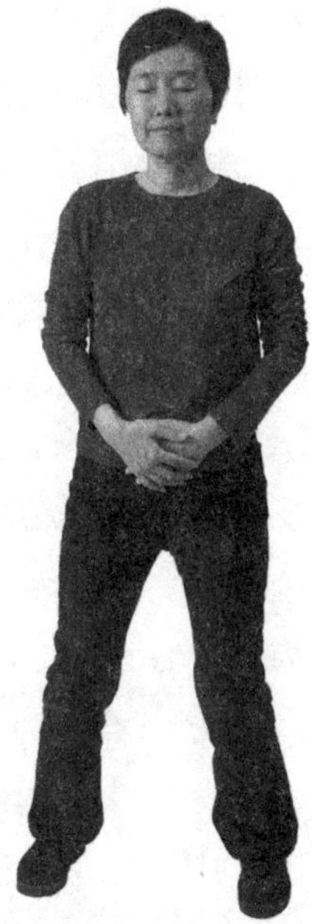

isn't deep enough. On the other hand, if the air you take in when inhaling primarily expands your abdomen, you probably know how to engage in abdominal breathing. Experiment now with different depths of inhaled breath and see where the air goes—to your chest or to your abdomen? Become more conscious of your habits in the days ahead.

Both fuller breathing and specific breathing exercises can bring many physiological and psychological benefits. First, they increase your intake of oxygen. This helps revitalize your cells, tissues, and organs and remove waste products. The fuller, more relaxed breathing associated with breath exercise also aids in moderating the function of your cerebral cortex, nervous system, and cardiovascular system. Proper breathing is also associated with lowering blood pressure. The organs in your abdominal cavity are gently massaged during breath work. Intentional breath exercises allow you to clear your mind and increase your awareness of the moment.

Breathing with a Smile

In the chapter on the Mindfulness Walk, we talked about intentionally putting a slight smile on your face to add joy to your life as you go through your daily walking routine. Here we will look at the combined qigong practice of both breathing and smiling to support your self-care regimen. This is called *Breathing with a Smile*, and its purpose is to open up the energy meridians in the body and promote general good health.

Perhaps you have heard about the powerful effect of laughter in promoting well-being and healing illness. The use of laughter became well-known through the 1979 book, *Anatomy of an Illness: As Perceived by the Patient* by Norman Cousins, former editor of *The Saturday Review.* Cousins astounded the medical world when he told his personal story of using laughter to recover from cancer. Since the book's publication, many researchers have studied and verified that laughter indeed adds many physical and psychological benefits to healing. Similarly, researchers have found that whether a smile is involuntary or not, it creates similar changes as laughter in the body. By choosing to wear a smile, you trigger some of the positive emotional and physiological changes you desire.

Moreover, adding abdominal breathing to a smile combines the benefits of both actions. Let's try *Breathing with a Smile*. Here's how to do it:

1. Choose a quiet, pleasant location and a comfortable chair. Sit silently with your feet on the ground. Rest your hands on your knees. Allow your body and mind to relax. As you let go of physical and mental tension, focus on your breathing. Your breathing should be relaxed, not forced. Breathe naturally down into your abdomen.
2. Close your eyes and begin to smile. Continue your abdominal breathing.
3. Picture in your mind something or someone that makes you smile. It could be a loved one or a good friend, or the thought of lily pads floating at one end of a beautiful pond. Keep smiling and your facial expression will soon begin to feel natural. Let go of any resistance you might feel.
4. Allow yourself to breathe deeply. Breathe and smile as you picture your lungs expanding with your breath. Breathe and smile as you visualize your shoulders relaxing. Breathe and smile as you think of your hands lying comfortably on your upper legs.

5. Let the various parts of your body relax as you focus on them with your breath and smile. Stay longer in any area that seems to be holding tension. Breathe gently and continue to smile. Let the tightness go. As the tension leaves your body, feel it being replaced with a loving, healing energy. Once your whole body is free of tension, you will begin to feel positive energy circulating in all areas as you keep breathing and smiling.
6. Enjoy the good feelings for several more minutes, and when you are ready, open your eyes. Sit still for a moment or two before rising.

At first, you might try this exercise for just five or ten minutes. Later, you can extend your practice to twenty minutes or a half hour. This exercise can be done once or twice a day, or just on the occasions when you need it.

Breathing for Healing and Energy

This breathing practice is used to build vital energy, support health and recovery, and reduce stress. It focuses on your inhalation and exhalation. You direct your inhalation into the Dan Tian, where your qi is stored (reminder: this is four finger widths below your navel). You then extend your exhalation for as long as you can, which aids with cleansing and creating a deep relaxation in the body. Here's how to do this exercise:

1. Find a quiet, comfortable location where you can sit and relax without being disturbed. Sit with your feet on the ground and legs separated. Rest your hands on your knees. Begin to relax as you take in a breath through your nose and down into your abdomen. Breathe out through your nose or mouth. Relax.
2. Inhale. Begin to sense a healing quality to the breath traveling down toward your Dan Tian. Feel the healing energy pour into your abdomen as your belly expands. Pause briefly at the end of the inhalation.
3. Now exhale slowly. As you breathe out through your mouth or nose, picture tensions and difficult emotions gently leaving your body. See this mixture easily dissolving into the air outside your body. As all of this is released, continue to feel a healing, energetic presence in your Dan Tian. Your exhalation should last longer than your inhalation.
4. Repeat a cycle of inhaling and exhaling. Feel healing energy enter your body and flow into

your Dan Tian. Exhale slowly to release more pressures and difficult emotions. Sense the positive energy from your Dan Tian begin to circulate into the rest of your body. Feel your body relaxing more and more as negative elements are released.

5. Continue the cycle of inhaling and exhaling for five minutes or more. When you've completed your breathing work, open your eyes. Sit quietly for a moment or two before rising.

This breathing practice can be helpful in getting in touch with the qi energy in your body. Breathing for healing and energy can be practiced for as long as a half hour. Mornings are a good time to work this practice into your routine.

The Basic Principles of a Qigong Healing Practice

Before we provide the instructions for the two qigong Immune Power Walks, here are some basic principles to keep in mind to enhance your practice.

Location

Qigong exercises can be performed either indoors or outside. Whichever you choose, find a quiet, pleasant area where the air is fresh. Outdoors, qigong is often practiced near trees or water. When you're inside, select a room with as much natural light and fresh air as possible, but avoid drafts or standing directly beneath a fan or by an air conditioner.

Correct Posture

Having good posture enables qi energy to flow more effectively throughout your body. As you stand, imagine that there is string attached to the top of your head that pulls you up and keeps your spine elongated. Make sure you are not slouching. Allow your shoulders to drop, and your chest is in a natural position, not caved in or puffed out. Your entire body is relaxed and firm.

Mental Receptiveness and Awareness

The mind is kept calm and concentrated during a qigong practice. This state of consciousness is similar to that of meditation. When your mind wanders and becomes preoccupied with daily concerns, notice that the mind has wandered, without any judgement, and simply redirect the mind to the sensations of the qigong movement.

As you do the qigong movements, you are aware of how your body moves. You observe your activity as you are involved in it. Yet you flow from one position to the next without tensing up in preparation for the subsequent moves.

Proper Breathing

As we have already emphasized, one of the keys to a healing qigong practice is to ensure that the body receives an adequate supply of oxygen. Through abdominal breathing and other special breath techniques, the body gains many benefits, including an enhancement in immune function and better regulation of its physiological systems. You may want to study the breathing aspects of the two Immune Power Walks separately from the movements. First, achieve a sense of competence in performing the qigong movements, then add in the suggested breathing patterns.

Ease of Movement

The qigong movements are made with a minimum of effort. No matter how difficult the position is, it is done efficiently and smoothly. This requires you to become conscious of how much effort is required, and then to do just that amount and no more or less.

Perseverance in Your Practice

When using qigong to enhance your health, it is best to be consistent and committed to a regular practice. Sporadic workouts don't produce sustained positive results. With a regular routine, you will see benefits build. Don't let the other demands in your life keep you from your qigong goals.

Empty Stomach

You should feel neither full nor hungry when you do qigong. If possible, practice on an empty stomach. If not, work the routines into your schedule about one to two hours after a meal. Digestion requires energy and detracts from the qi that is available to move throughout your body during your workout.

Body Sensations

You may notice various sensations in your body during a qigong practice, such as a warming or cooling feeling. This is not unusual, so do not be concerned.

Ending the Practice

End each session smoothly and calmly, not abruptly. This helps maintain your flow of qi energy throughout the day.

Preparatory Exercise for the Immune Power Walks

The following exercise is recommended before doing either of the two Immune Power Walks presented here. The goal is to enter a state of relaxation, both physically and mentally. The exercise also produces adjustments in your breathing that facilitate calmness and help to oxygenate your body. Note: your eyes should remain closed throughout the entire exercise once you have learned how to do it.

1. Stand in a relaxed manner and quiet your mind. Your feet should be about shoulder-width apart, with your knees slightly bent. Your center of gravity is in your lower abdomen.
2. Your arms should hang naturally at your sides, perpendicular to the ground. Relax your shoulders. Remain in this position for a few minutes as you relax further.

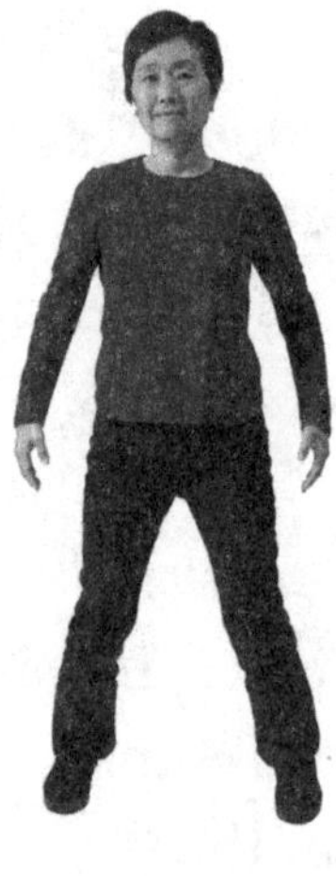

3. Place your left hand on your abdomen with the palm facing your Dan Tian energy center (about four finger widths below

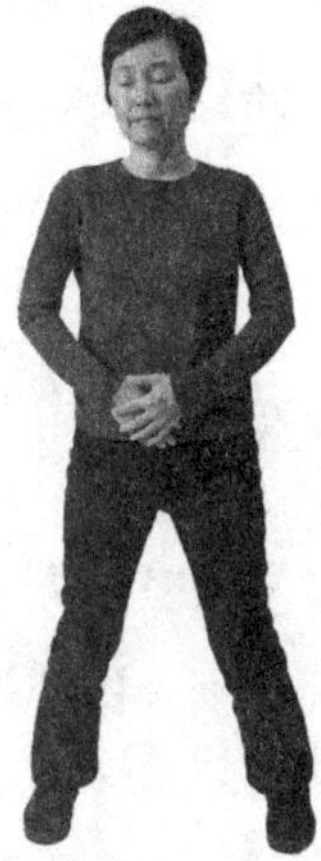

your navel). Next place the palm of your right hand over your left.

4. Open your mouth slightly. Inhale, breathing deeply through the nose into your abdomen, while lowering your body by bending the knees. At the end of the inhalation, exhale slowly. Only when you have finished exhaling should you raise your body to the initial position. Repeat this breathing pattern three times.
5. Next, lower your arms, raise your elbows, and invert your hands so the backs are facing each other in front of your body. Then move your hands away from your body, as if you were parting water. Rotate your hands so that the palms are facing each other at your sides.

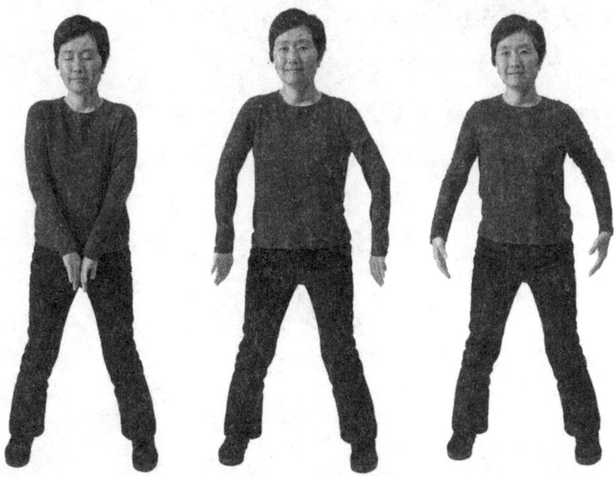

6. Now push the water back towards the center of your body, as if you were holding a small balloon. Then bring your hands back together, palms facing one another, and fold them gently on your abdomen.
7. Open and close your hands several times, then repeat the sequence of hand movements described in Steps 5 and 6.
8. When you are done, rest for a moment with your eyes closed. Allow your hands to hang relaxed at your sides.

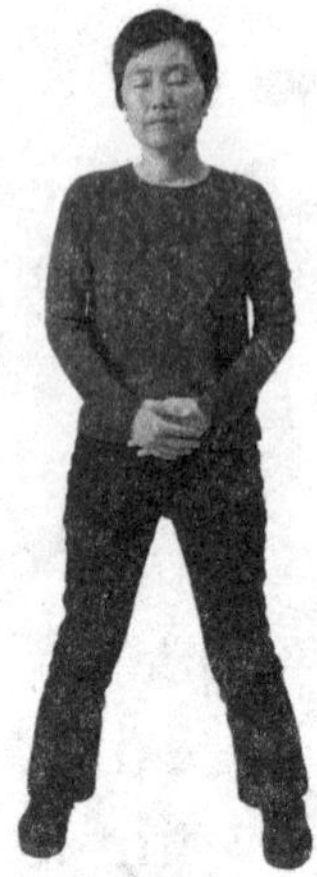

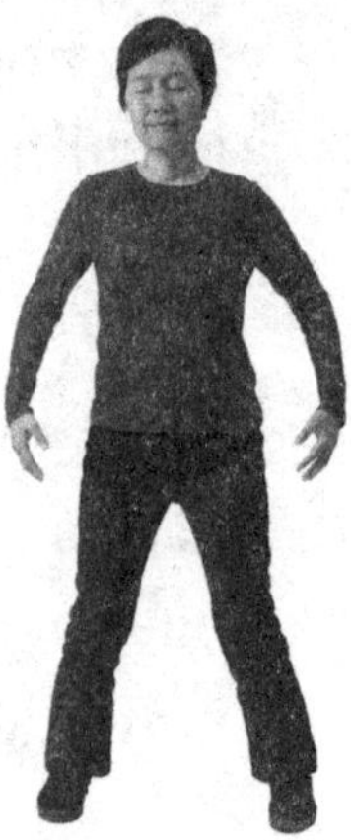

This exercise prepares you to move onto one of the Immune Power Walks.

Immune Power Walk 1: The Wind Breath Walk

This walk serves as the foundation for many of the other styles of qigong walks derived from Guo Lin's work. It synchronizes movement, breathing, weight distribution, and hand positioning. The Wind Breath Walk exercises the entire body, strengthens your qi energy, and can be used to address various ailments. You'll find the walk easy to learn. It can be practiced in a nearby park, your backyard, or in a large room. Begin by closing your eyes once you have learned how to do this walk.

1. Close your eyes and stand in the same manner as you did for the preparatory exercise. Your mind and body should be relaxed, and your feet about shoulder-width apart. Bend your knees slightly and relax your shoulders.
2. Slowly open your eyes. Continue to relax.
3. Inhale as you step forward with your left foot. *All* of your weight should still reside on the right leg. Allow the base of your left heel to hit the floor, with your toes facing up. As you step forward, turn your head and

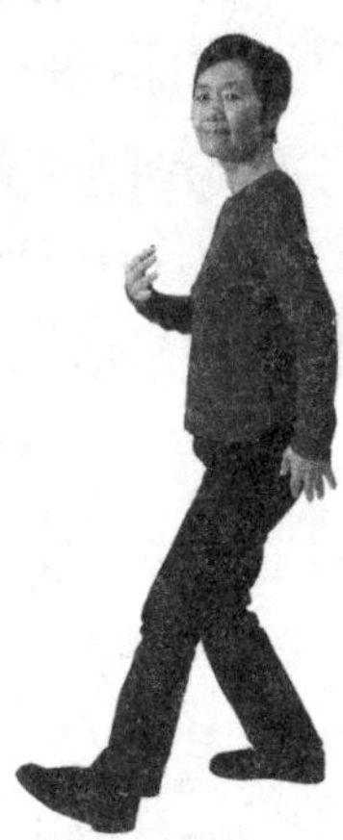

twist your spine to the left without straining, while swinging your right arm forward in front of you until your palm is facing your sternum or heart in a relaxed fashion. Your left hand goes back past your hip as if you were reaching for a tool on a tool belt. Exhale and make sure you empty your lungs.

4. Shift your weight to your left foot as it flattens out and step forward with your right foot. Turn your neck and torso to the right, which stimulates the neural outlets from the cervical spine, and sniff in through your nose twice as in the Vitality Walk. As your left foot flattens out, sniff out once. Step with your right foot, heel landing first, toes up. Move your left hand in front of your heart. Your right hand should go back and rest near your hip. Turn your neck toward the right, and sniff in through your nose twice. As the right foot flattens out, sniff out once.

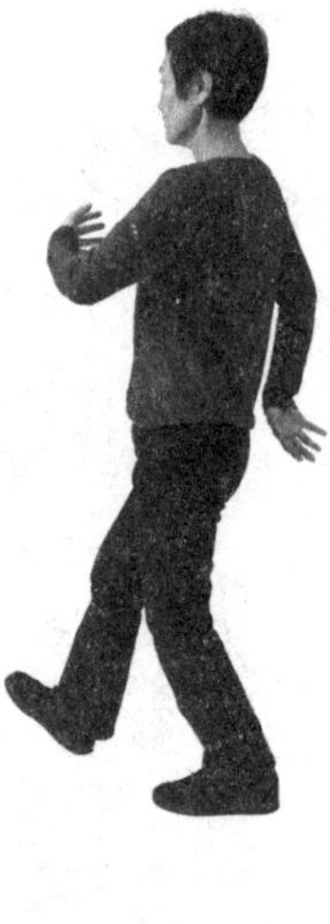

5. Repeat the movement sequences for the desired period. When you're finished, walk naturally for a minute or two.

When learning the Wind Breath Walk, you may want to perfect your movements before trying the special breathing exercise. Once you are proficient at the walk, add in the in-in-out breathing pattern to harmonize with the steps.

If you are using the Wind Breath Walk for conditioning and prevention, it is usually practiced twice a day, once in the morning and then again in the evening. You can start out with about five minutes of practice at a time, and gradually move up to ten, twenty, or thirty minutes of practice. After a while, you might do the walk for as long as an hour.

After you are comfortable with a ten-minute practice, you can learn the advanced walk.

Immune Power Walk 2: Advanced Immune Power Walk

The Advanced Immune Power Walk is similar to the Wind Breath Walk, but it has slightly different characteristics. First, the breathing takes place over three steps of the foot. Also, you will move slightly to the side rather than straight ahead. In addition, the movement is a little faster than in the first walk to accommodate the spreading of the breathing pattern over more steps.

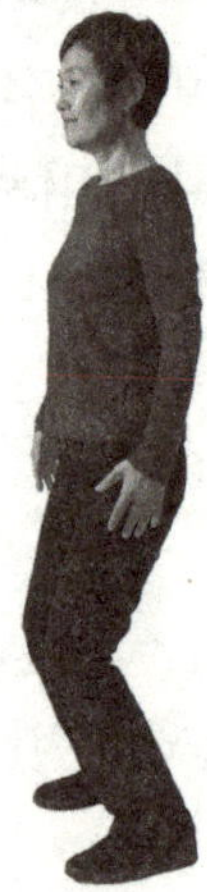

1. Close your eyes and stand as you did for the preparatory exercise. Relax your mind and body. Your feet should be about shoulder-width apart, with knees slightly bent. Your shoulders are relaxed.
2. Slowly open your eyes. Continue to relax.
3. Shift all of your weight to the right side. Begin to step forward and to the side with your left foot at about a 45-degree angle. Move your left arm back to your hip like you are reaching for a tool on a tool belt. Rotate your upper body slightly to the left, as you swing your right arm in front of you (palm facing your abdomen). Sniff in once.

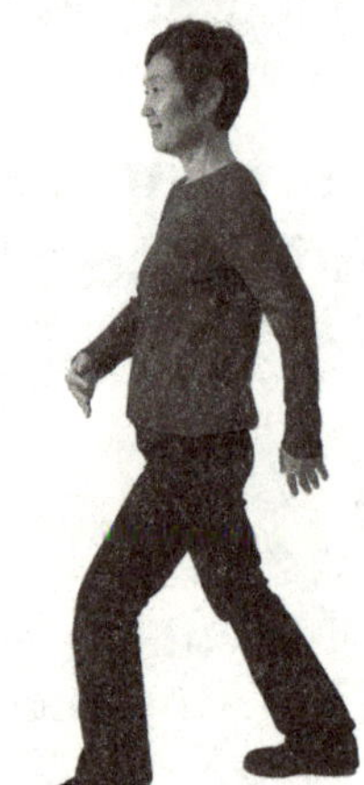

4. Reverse the movement by shifting your weight to the right side. Begin to step to the side with your right foot. Move

your right arm down and back toward your hip.

5. Swing your left arm up toward your abdomen (palm facing in). Rotate your upper body, head, and neck slightly to the right. Sniff in again.
6. Repeat this three-step sequence as you alternate the breath every three steps. When you're finished, walk naturally for a minute or two.

As with the Wind Breath Walk, you may find it easier to master the movements before adding them to the special breathing pattern.

This walk is usually done twice a day for optimal results—once in the morning and then in the evening—for those who are seeking to heal from an illness. Start with about five minutes and work up gradually to a ten-, twenty-, or thirty-minute practice.

The two walks can be done in a combined practice, splitting the time evenly, or moving back and forth with five minutes of each walk. In time, you may want to do an hour of the Advanced Immune Power Walk by itself, or an hour combining the two exercises, depending on your goals.

The Future of Medical Qigong

Qigong practices for health and well-being have been growing in popularity in many parts of the world, including the United States. The study of the medical benefits of qigong is sure to undergo further research. At this time, researchers have identified numerous positive effects on the body and mind, but its full potential is yet unknown. For now, we know that it offers many physical and mental benefits, and we believe that your qigong practice will be a positive activity to add to your life. Like learning a musical instrument, keep at the practice, increase in small increments, and be consistent.

Week 5
The Tai Chi Animal Walks for Balance

What is the aim of Tai Chi Chuan practice? Health and vitality and eternal spring.

—Wu Yu Xiang

Tai Chi is one of the most widely recognized and popular of the Chinese martial arts, practiced worldwide. Tai chi is anchored in the Chinese philosophy of Daoism (pronounced dowism), which seeks a harmonious way of life and recognizes the importance of nature. The term *tai chi* was shortened from "tai chi chuan" (pronounced *tie jee chuwan)* which literally means "supreme ultimate fist."

In practice, tai chi is a sophisticated sequence of roughly 108 movements based on the qigong principle of involving the whole body in physical coordination. The tai chi movements we have chosen—the tai chi Cat Walk, the Golden Rooster Walk, and the Bear Spirit Walk (not to be confused with Yoga Bear Walk)—involve movements mimicked from animals, as are many of the motions in tai chi and other martial arts. For centuries, martial artists studied animal motions and incorporated their fighting strategies and movements into human practices.

Tai chi was originally developed as a fighting practice for combat, emphasizing strength, speed, and flexibility. However, in the last century, tai chi has received more attention as a health-supporting practice. Ironically, one reason for this was the introduction of firearms to the battlefields of China in the twentieth century. This caused a loss of interest in tai chi as a fighting technique. Many martial arts practitioners have developed their arts for other benefits besides combat, especially health, with slower, more fluid, softer movements that show off the human body's suppleness and strength. While practicing tai chi moves, it is said that you bend your body gently like "bamboo in the wind."

Tai chi's popularity in the West, especially in the US, has grown tremendously over the past decades and continues to expand. Before the turn of the millennium, someone performing tai chi in a public park in the early morning was unusual in the West.

There are many reasons for the spread of tai chi's popularity, but perhaps the most prevalent is that the art is revered for its ability to help develop amazing balance skills and a keen awareness of the body as it moves through space. In fact, tai chi is fast becoming a regular component of more and more balance-training programs for older adults, who face grave consequences should they fall, such as broken legs, arms, and hips, which then lead to debilitating lifetime walking problems.

We believe that acquiring balance skills is important for anyone at any age, so that is our purpose in teaching these three tai chi walks. By doing these practices, you will learn to maintain balance while gracefully performing a series of physical moves that alternate between inaction and motion.

Tai chi views this relationship of inactivity and motion through the principles of yin and yang—the two polar opposites in Chinese tradition. These elements complement each other and create a natural balance. As you learn to move from stillness to motion and back to stillness to do a series of moves in the tai chi walks, your awareness of how your body makes such transitions will increase.

The neo-Confucian Chou Tun-I (1017–1073) was one of the first to write about how stillness and movement relate:

> The Great Ultimate [tai chi] through movement generates yang. When its activity reaches its limit, it becomes tranquil. Through tranquility, the Great Ultimate generates yin. When tranquility reaches its limit, activity begins again. So movement and tranquility alternate and become the root of each other, giving rise to the distinction of yin and yang, and the two modes are thus established.[1]

There are many other benefits to practicing the tai chi movements, including increasing flexibility, reducing stress, slowing the aging process, helping with arthritis, and achieving better overall health. We will explain these benefits in this chapter, but first you might be interested in knowing how the practice of tai chi developed over time.

The Origins of Tai Chi

The history of tai chi is rich and deep. Its origins are commonly associated with the story of a tall, bearded Daoist monk, Chang San-feng, who lived in the thirteenth century. It is said that Chang developed the unique style that has become tai chi while living alone in the misty and craggy Wu Dang Mountains in China. In one version of the legend, Chang created the tai chi animal moves after watching a snake battling a crane. He was impressed that the weaker animal could defeat the stronger one by exhausting his opponent through yielding. Chang decided to create a new martial arts form combining the fighting skills he had previously learned with movements from animals and nature. These movements included those of the snake, as well as natural elements such as water, wind, and clouds. The result was tai chi.

It is not known whether Chang San-feng truly existed, but it does seem clear that tai chi originated centuries ago. Over time, different families in China developed their own versions of tai chi. Here is a brief overview of four of the major styles as background for your understanding of tai chi. (Note: the three practices we teach you in this chapter reflect a combination of styles of our own.)

Chen Style: The family generally considered the ancestor of modern tai chi can be traced back to an army officer, Chen Want Ting, in the seventeenth century. Chen synthesized tai chi movements in the 1670s, based on a training manual for military troops written a century earlier. His tai chi incorporated clarity of consciousness, internal power, and deep breathing. Fast and hard movements are mixed with softer moves, and the positions use a low stance.

Yang Style: In the early part of the nineteenth century, a descendant of Chen Wang Ting taught the Chen style to an exceptional martial arts student from outside the family, Yang Luchan (1799–1872). Yang then combined his earlier martial arts studies with what he learned from the Chen style, and his movements became known as the Yang style. The Yang style is considered the most prevalent of the schools of tai chi as the movements are easy to learn, graceful, and accessible to older adults and those with health concerns.

Wu Style: Second in popularity today is the Wu school of tai chi. The stance for the Wu style is high, and its approach to tai chi is soft, relaxed, and straightforward, with slow, compact movements performed close to the body.

Sun Style: This style arose by combining elements from two other internal martial arts—Ba Gua (which you will learn about in chapter 6) and Xing-I—and incorporated them with tai chi. The Sun style is the most modern of the various schools, blending the Ba Gua approach to stepping, the leg and waist movements of Xing-I, and the gentleness of tai chi. The stance for the Sun style is high, making it accessible for students who have difficulty crouching.

* * *

The Health Benefits of Tai Chi

We have already discussed many of the physical, emotional, and mental health benefits of walking in chapter 1, and the practice of doing tai chi alone or as part of your daily walk contributes to those benefits. In fact, tai chi has become one of the most popular martial arts due to its healthful effects on the human body and spirit. A 2022 Harvard Health article stated,

> Tai Chi is often described as "*meditation* in motion," but it might well be called *medication* in motion. There is growing evidence that this mind-body practice, which originated in China as a martial art, has value in treating or preventing many health problems. And you can get started even if you aren't in top shape or the best of health.[2]

In fact, many people begin tai chi because of an illness or injury, and it is increasingly credited as a major factor in their recovery. Here is a brief review of the preventive health benefits you can derive from tai chi.

Muscle Strength

It is often accepted that becoming weaker, stiffer, and less mobile is a natural and unavoidable part of the aging process. However, recent research findings indicate that aging does not necessarily cause less mobility; rather it is a sedentary lifestyle that creates the conditions for becoming weak and stiff as you age. Numerous studies confirm that regular exercise slows down the aging process, helps retain muscle mass, and preserves strength.

More specifically, a large body of carefully conducted research has demonstrated that tai chi helps adults, especially older adults, to keep moving and stay in shape. The tai chi Cat Walk, the Golden Rooster Walk, and the Bear Spirit Walk taught in this chapter strengthen the legs and improve both lower-body and upper-body strength, similar to resistance training.

Balance

Tai chi has proven more effective than many common forms of exercise for developing balance skills. The movements in the three animal practices we teach are designed to focus constant attention on your balance. As the body continually changes form during the movements of the walks, it taps into different muscular dynamics and proprioceptors, having the ability to sense the body movement in space, thus improving balance. The skills you develop when performing the practices naturally carry over into your everyday life. They help you move with more grace, give you confidence against the fear of falling, and enable you to regain your balance quickly if you happen to trip or stumble.

A key element in how tai chi helps your balance is that it improves your sense of your body in space. This is a function of the sensory neurons in your inner ear and your ability to coordinate your location in space with muscle control to stay upright.

Flexibility and Body Toning

Generally, our physical body tone is at its peak in our twenties. As we move into our fifties and sixties, we often lose our toning gradually, and afterward more rapidly if we don't take measures to exercise our muscles and stay flexible. A tai chi practice is a way to gently exercise the joints and major muscle groups. Joints remain flexible and muscles get stronger—especially in the legs. People who have practiced tai chi into their sixties, seventies, and eighties are still able to do the exercises without difficulty, having preserved their strength. There are currently well-known tai chi teachers in their nineties and even over a hundred.

The Tai Chi Animal Walks promote both strength and agility in the lower muscles and joints. While doing the walks, the way you carry the weight of your body changes continuously. If you do one of the Tai Chi Animal Walks consistently, you will notice a development in both muscle size and the strength of your legs. Maintaining leg strength is important for staying fit. As a Chinese saying expresses it: "The legs are the mirror of one's health."

Help with Rheumatoid Arthritis, Osteoarthritis, and Back Pain

People with rheumatoid arthritis face a conundrum. If your joints are full of pain and stiffness, you don't feel much like exercising. However, if you don't exercise, your ability to move will likely become even more limited.

Tai chi is one activity that more and more doctors and physical therapists recommend for people with arthritis. It offers all three components that medical professionals look for in a therapeutic exercise program—flexibility training, muscle strengthening, and fitness benefits.

A number of research studies have correlated tai chi with improvements for people with arthritis. In one systematic review of three clinical studies involving patients with arthritis found that the effects of tai chi in conjunction with education and stretching exercises versus education and stretching alone showed greater improvements in the variables of mood, depression and functionality.[3] Other benefits that arthritis sufferers experience when they do tai chi are better posture and better energy, although these benefits apply to everyone who practices tai chi.

Dr. Paul Lam, a family physician in Australia, even developed the Tai Chi for Arthritis program. A tai chi teacher for more than fifty years and founder of the Tai Chi for Health Institute, Dr. Lam initially became interested in this exercise form when he himself suffered from arthritis. Many of the people in Lam's program experienced relief from arthritis symptoms by doing tai chi. The US Centers for

Disease Control and Prevention recommend Dr. Lam's Tai Chi for Arthritis for Fall Prevention program, as does the National Council on Aging, and the Arthritis Foundation. (Note: if you have arthritis and feel any concerns about performing a tai chi–related routine, consult your health professional before getting started.)

As for osteoarthritis, a study by researchers at Tufts Medical Center in Boston found that tai chi could reduce the pain and physical impairment of people with severe knee osteoarthritis. And the American College of Physicians recommended the use of tai chi in their 2017 treatment guidelines. They cite that research shows that the slow, gentle movements of tai chi, along with deep breathing, helps ease back pain by strengthening the muscles in the abdomen and pelvic areas which support the lower back. As part of the US Department of Veteran Affairs' Whole Health Initiative, tai chi is taught at VA centers across the United States.

Stress Reduction

Stress is a part of life, and so it is hard to avoid. Some stress is positive, such as when we are pushed to be productive by a deadline. But the level of stress most of us face appears to be on the rise. The 2024 results of the American Psychiatric Association's annual mental health poll indicate a growing sense of anxiety among US adults. In 2024, 43 percent of adults reported feeling more anxious than in prior years.

Unfortunately, it is now known that the constant pressure of stress affects our health. Health researchers have traced many diseases that are brought on or worsened by stress. These include high blood pressure, coronary heart disease, cancer, chronic pain, gastrointestinal problems, type 2 diabetes, headaches, back pain, and skin disorders.

The way you respond to stress is actually the key. Given a stressful situation, you might respond calmly and evenly, not allowing the stress to exacerbate the situation. Or you might react with anxiety and tension, which tightens your muscles, releases potentially cell-harming hormones in your blood, and puts your body into the fight-or-flight response mode. Researchers now know that those people who can stay calm through stress management techniques can lower their health risks.

This is where tai chi practices can help you. The Tai Chi Animal Walks are powerful stress reducers. One reason is that great concentration is required to do these tai chi movements smoothly and gracefully. Your focused concentration enables you to take a break from whatever causes you to feel tension and anxiety. Your mind is simply too focused to be stressed.

A regular tai chi practice also helps you become more aware of your body, so you can recognize when it is beginning to react to the stressors in your life. Tai chi teaches you to feel when your muscles are tensing up, and even when your internal body processes are reacting to stress and going into the fight or flight mode. You learn how to scan your body and pinpoint where you are holding stress so you can release it. You also learn how to relax and voluntarily let go of body tension, so that you can go on with your day relaxed, refreshed, and alert.

Lower Blood Pressure

In addition, practicing tai chi creates many positive physiological changes originating in the parasympathetic nervous system. As part of this response, your heart rate slows down and your blood pressure decreases. Pain associated with muscle tension and stress is often reduced as the body relaxes. The departure of pain can also help you feel less anxiety.

One large study in China documents the effectiveness of a regular tai chi practice in lowering blood pressure. The study involved 342 adults aged eighteen to sixty-five years with prehypertension, and was conducted between July 2019 and January 2022 at two public hospitals in China. Researchers randomly assigned participants to one of two interventions in hour-long sessions four times per week. About half participated in supervised aerobic exercise, including jogging, brisk walking, cycling, and stair-climbing. The other half practiced tai chi. The results found that a twelve-month tai chi intervention was more effective than the aerobic exercise in reducing blood pressure.[4]

Such studies demonstrate that you don't have to exhaust yourself with strenuous exercise in order to lower your blood pressure. Light exercise, such as tai chi, can help reduce blood pressure just as effectively as (or even more effectively than) rigorous workouts such as running.

Cardiovascular Benefits

Tai chi is a form of low-intensity cardiopulmonary exercise. As such, it can assist in preventing heart disease and even in reversing it. During a tai chi practice, your heart rate increases at a moderate and steady pace rather than in bursts like in aerobic exercise. With tai chi, the heart is not overburdened. You receive the exercise benefits to your cardiovascular system without excessively stressing your body. Tai chi is a cardiotonic, rather than a cardio stressor. It gives your circulatory system a gentle workout.

Often those who have high blood pressure also experience hardening of the arteries. Tai chi can be helpful here, too. Because of the design of the moves, muscles smoothly contract and relax. Arteries and veins are thus massaged, resulting in more effective contractions and expansions and smoother blood flow, which takes away waste products produced in the muscles. With regular tai chi practice, a buildup of cholesterol is less likely, and even cholesterol already clogging the walls of veins and arteries can be diminished with the increased blood flow.

Stroke Recovery

A stroke is a medical emergency when a blood vessel in the brain becomes blocked or ruptures, impairing blood and oxygen flow to brain tissue. This can result in paralysis, loss of muscle movement and coordination issues, loss of speech, memory loss, cognitive difficulties, changes in behavior, and emotional problems.

Some research shows that tai chi can help stroke victims recover faster. One twelve-week study conducted in China involved 160 participants who were randomly divided into two groups. One group practiced a form of seated tai chi while the other group had a standard stroke rehabilitation program. At the end of the study, the tai chi participants had improved hand and arm function, better balance control, wider shoulder range of motion, and improved mental health and quality of life compared to those patients in the standard rehabilitation program.[5]

Immune Function Support

Research indicates that regular exercise, including tai chi, can reward you with improved immunity. During exercise, blood flow increases, and cell metabolism is thus raised. The production of endorphins—the hormones that make you feel good—is sped up. Endorphins also have a beneficial effect on immune function.

A 2020 systematic review of nineteen randomized controlled research studies involving 1,686 participants to explore the effects of tai chi and qigong on the immune system showed that tai chi had a statistically significant effect of increasing the levels of immune cells.[6]

By contrast, some research in the past found that intense physical exertion can decrease immune function. One study noted, for example, that more than ninety minutes of high-intensity endurance exercise made athletes susceptible to illness for up to seventy-two hours after the exercise session.[7] This was attributed to the fact that during intense physical exertion, certain hormones were produced that temporarily lowered immunity.

Origins of the Tai Chi Animal Walks

It is possible that the imitation of animals traces back thousands of years to a famous medical doctor in China, Hua Tuo, during the Han dynasty (206 BCE to 200 AD). An expert in acupuncture, gynecology, pediatrics, and surgery, and an innovator of herbal medicines, he is credited with creating what became known as the Five Animal Frolics. His inspiration came from observing the movements of various animals and concluding that these movements enhanced the animals' overall health. He focused on five animals—tigers, deer, bears, monkeys, and birds. Each one had its own characteristic movements which Hua Tuo sought to emulate, both physically and mentally, to capture the animal's spirit. The physical movements tried to emulate the courage of the tiger; the serenity and poise of the deer; the solidity of the bear; the nimbleness and dexterity of the monkey; and the swiftness and grace of the bird. Hua Tuo's movements were thought to strengthen the muscles and bones, improve the circulation of qi in the body, and prevent or cure disease. Although there are no written documents or drawings of the Five Animal Frolics, the Cat Walk, the Golden Rooster Walk, and Bear Spirit Walk are descendants of Hua Tuo's movements.

The Tai Chi Animal Walks

We will present three basic practices in this chapter—the Cat Walk, the Golden Rooster Walk, and the Bear Spirit Walk. In these movements, the sequence is repeated to create a walking-like experience. Here are ten basic tai chi principles that will help you do these movements correctly.

Balance and Body Awareness

In tai chi, balance is achieved through a heightened level of sensitivity to your body's movements. In fact, the ideal standard in tai chi states that the practitioner should learn to distribute tension and relaxation throughout the body. This is the high level of awareness and connection to your body that you want to develop through an extended tai chi practice.

In achieving a state of physical balance, the lower body is instrumental because it supports the rest of you. The upper body is lighter and softer, with the shoulders relaxed. You should feel like you are floating upward. Focus on and breathe through any tensions you feel that initially challenge your efforts to stay comfortably in balance. In time, the tightness will ease.

Slow Movement

Move slowly, giving the activity your total attention. Aim to make your tempo consistent throughout your entire session. A slow rate allows your body to remain relaxed and your muscles flexible and resilient. At this pace, you do not waste your energy nor totally expend it too early. Also, the slow speed helps you control the movements and adds to your body consciousness. You want to enjoy exploring the intricacies of each move.

Lightness

There's a story about the Golden Rooster Walk that states that it was devised by a teacher who had reached an advanced level of ability to be light on his feet during movement. Stepping on an uncovered manhole in the street, he did not fall in but merely compensated by stepping forward over it with his other foot. His ability to be light was complemented by his extraordinary awareness of his surroundings, so that he sensed the lack of support under his foot before falling into the hole in the street!

Lightness in tai chi is achieved by not being forceful in creating motion, but letting it flow naturally and continuously. In fact, tai chi involves a circular flow that supports lightness and creates soft, even, smooth movements.

Awareness of Gravity

In doing the Tai Chi Animal Walks, you will need to reawaken your awareness of how gravity pulls on your body. You will want to become more aware of your biomechanics—the feel, structure, and workings of your body. To enhance your awareness, you must first sense your body weight in space. As you move, try to feel gravity's force as a friction created between your body and the atmosphere around it. This sensation is somewhat like swimming or moving in water.

Remember that in water, if you move slowly and naturally, you make progress easily. Have an image in your mind of a graceful, continuous motion, like the flight of a bird. While doing the Tai Chi Animal

Walks, movements will seem like they are about to stop, but they don't; they flow one into the next.

Awareness of the Ground

A counterbalance to gravity is the support we receive from the ground. This is a solid and limiting force that offers support by resisting gravity's efforts to pull us downward. In your mind, compare the experience of walking on the ground or floor to stepping into a pool of water. The ground helps you stabilize your movements.

Whole-Body Coordination

As you move your legs in the Tai Chi Animal Walks, your whole body will work together in total coordination. Initially, you will likely be conscious of particular areas of your body, but with time you will begin to sense how the whole body works as a unit. Also, each step in the sequence of moves should flow smoothly into the next.

Fullness versus Emptiness

Tai chi looks at a sequence of movements in terms of the parts of the body that are active (full) or inactive (empty). Yang is associated with activeness, while yin is tied to stillness. These concepts are also referred to as substantial and insubstantial. Thinking in these terms, you should keep in mind that the empty (inactive) part of the body is actually never completely devoid of energy. There is always a certain mix of both activity and stillness. These concepts are used to explain weight distribution in various moves. The weighted part is yang (active or full); the section of the body that isn't handling the weight is yin (inactive or empty).

Breathing

Most of us breathe too shallowly in our everyday lives, because we fail to breathe fully into our abdomen. Abdominal breathing is especially important when performing the movements of tai chi. Initially, as you're learning the Tai Chi Animal Walks, breathe in a normal way, but make sure that the air flows all the way down into your abdomen. Do this in a gentle way. Allow your mind and body to relax as you breathe easily in and out.

As you become comfortable with the movements, study the mode of breathing pattern explained next. Although you will initially breathe very automatically when you begin practicing tai chi, practice the following style so you can be consciously aware of it. As you perform the breathing pattern, be aware of the air moving in and out of your body. See it through visualization.

- *Natural Mode.* Natural mode breathing is cooling and calming. It has yin energy. It stimulates relaxation of the body and slows the heart rate. In this style, the main focus is on the inhalation. A goal is to train your sides and back to move with your abdomen while you breathe. This should be accomplished in a relaxed manner. Do not force air in a severe way into your body. Before working with your back and sides, concentrate on gentle, deep abdominal breathing. Expand your back and sides to deepen your breathing.

Breathing is a critical component of relaxing and developing body awareness. Once you become proficient at this breathing style, you might enjoy practicing a short session of conscious breathing before and after your tai chi practices. As you do the Tai Chi Animal Walks, you will be more aware of when your body is shifting from one mode to the other. With practice, you will be able to enhance your body's natural process.

Every part of the body needs an ample supply of oxygen in order to perform well. Short sessions of conscious breathing help support good health as well as recovery from illness.

Note: if you decide to explore tai chi at a more advanced level, you will be trained in how to coordinate movement and breathing. The basic principles are as follows:

- Open on exhalation and close on inhalation
- Rise on inhalation and fall on exhalation
- Inhale during defensive movements and exhale during attacking

Calmness in Activity

In martial arts—such as karate, judo, and tae kwon do—energetic movements and the outward exertion of force can heighten the emotions that the performer experiences. In contrast, tai chi emphasizes a tranquil spirit during movement, and the nature of the fluid tai chi movements themselves is calm. Concentration on the intended result quiets the mind.

The Tai Chi Animal Walks

The three practices you are about to learn can be performed in a backyard, park, or large open room.

Start by practicing the tai chi Cat Walk for two or three minutes and then slowly build up to ten minutes. When you can do ten minutes of the tai chi Cat Walk, try the Golden Rooster Walk, and then the Bear Spirit Walk. Once you learn the three practices, you can do one or a combination of three for about thirty minutes at a time. If you enjoy the practice, you can do the practices for thirty minutes twice a day.

The Cat Walk

The tai chi Cat Walk is an excellent tai chi movement for improving balance skills. The pattern of footwork is very important in a tai chi practice. It was first used in the Yang style. The founder's grandson, Yang Cheng Fu, wrote in his book *The Practice of Taijiquan* that "the legs should be based upon Yin [emptiness] and Yang [fullness] with the legs rising and lowering like a cat."

In *Essentials of Free-Sparring*, Yu Xiang wrote that the performer should "step like a walking cat and issue power like weaving silk." The reference to silk weaving means that you should move in a slow, even, and flowing manner.

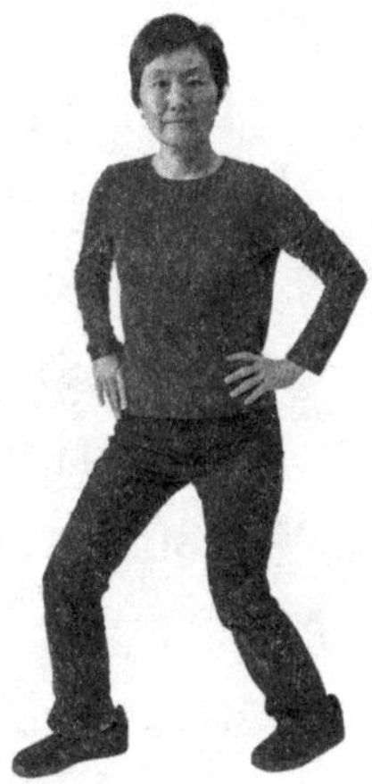

1. Begin by assuming what is considered a right bow stance. In this position, the right leg is forward and bent at the knee (but not beyond your toes). The lower half of the right leg is perpendicular to the ground (in other words, straight up and down). The left leg is straight back behind you, with a slight bend. Your entire weight is on your right leg (making it "full"), and your left leg has no weight (making it "empty"). The toes of your right foot are pointing straight ahead, while the toes of your left foot are at a 45-degree angle toward the left. Your hands are resting on the upper part of your hips at belt level (the iliac crest).
2. Relax into this form and check your positioning. Your upper body should be erect. Make sure your back is straight and your chin slightly dropped. Imagine a straight line drawn from the top of your head down the middle of

your lower body. Picture a bowl of water being balanced on your head to achieve the proper alignment. (See the photo on page 129.)

3. Now sink your waist down and rotate toward the right as your right hip also sinks and turns slightly outward. Lift the toes of your right foot and rotate them outward at a 45-degree angle toward the right. Don't move your right heel and maintain your nearly 100 percent weight distribution on the right foot. These actions occur at virtually the same time.
4. Slowly pick up your left foot and bring it through to the front. Use your left hip joint to bring the left leg forward in a relaxed manner. Your left leg should be slightly bent but held under your body as you pull it forward. Your toes should be pointed downward and slightly above the ground. As the left leg passes the right, it should be bent, with the bottom half hanging directly toward the ground. Straighten your left leg before you gently bring down your heel. The toes of your left foot should be pointing up in a natural way. Bring the foot through, ending with your whole left foot on the floor.

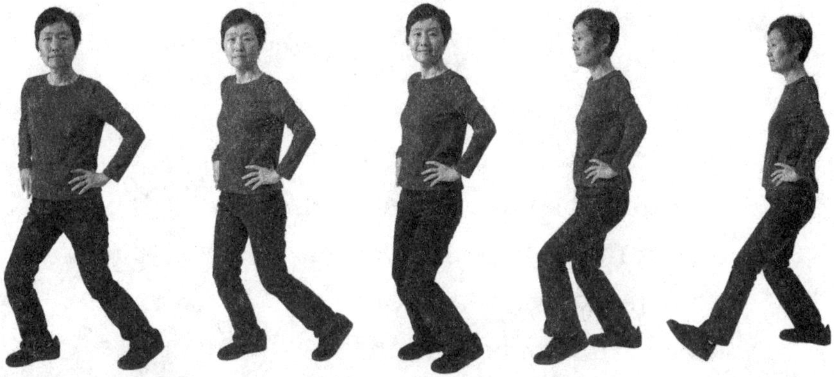

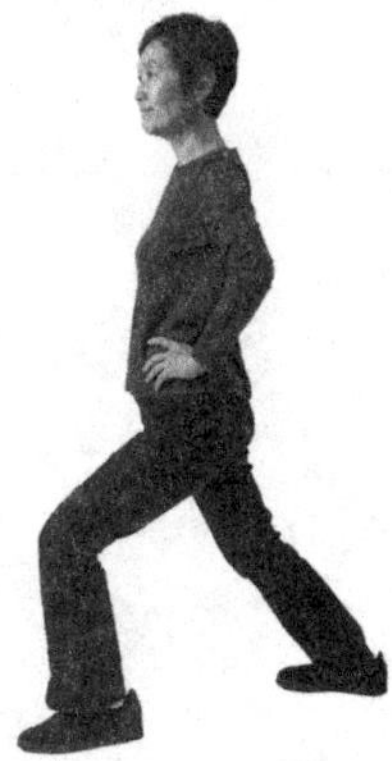

5. As you lower the toes of your left foot to the ground, your right leg straightens behind you. Continue leaning forward on your left leg until you are standing in a left bow stance that mirrors the right bow stance you started with. Your weight is now all on your left leg (making it full), and the right leg has no weight (making it empty).
6. Continue these moves for the duration of your walk, five to ten minutes ideally.
7. Stand in the "Wu Ji" position for a minute. This position, also known as Standing Like a Pole, is widely used in martial arts because it helps with centering yourself and clearing your mind. To stand in this position, stand as still as you can, feet shoulder-width apart.

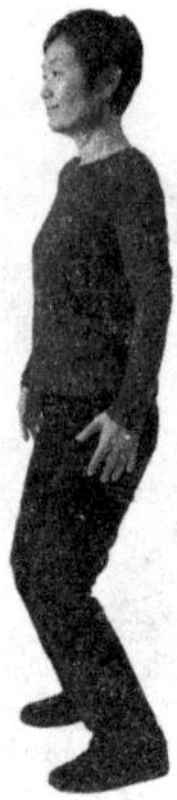

Gaze out in front of you with a soft focus. Allow your arms to relax but leave a small amount of space between your arms and your body. Elongate your neck and bend your knees slightly. Feel a sense of elongation in your spinal column. Inhale and exhale in a relaxed manner.

The Golden Rooster Walk

The Golden Rooster Walk (a.k.a., The Golden Rooster Stands on One Leg) is more advanced than the Cat Walk. The movement sequence is used in many forms of tai chi with slight alterations. The description comes from the Sun family style. In each family variation of tai chi, individual developers added their own insights to the performance of the moves. There are even variations within the family styles. In the case of the Golden Rooster Walk, one difference is that in some forms, the elbow is allowed to rest on the knee when the leg is raised. When you are new to this walk, this may help you maintain the form. However, it is better not to touch your elbow and thigh so that your back and spine can remain straight.

To do the Golden Rooster Walk, begin as follows:

1. Bend your knees and assume a half-squatting position. Shift your weight to your right leg (full). Lower your arms, with your fingers pointing downward. Your left leg stays behind you and is bent at the knee. Your left heel is slightly raised to allow this bend. Your right leg is now just slightly in front of your body.

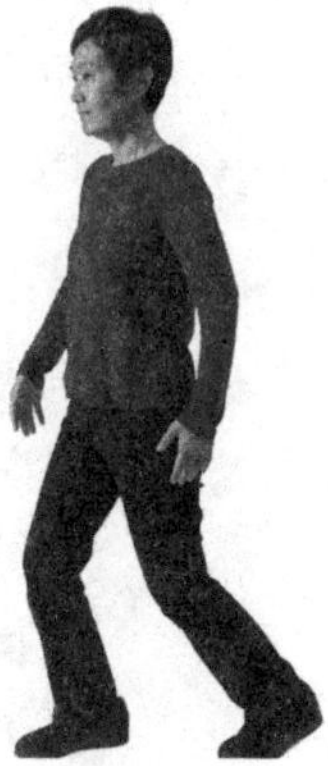

2. Now straighten your right leg slightly as it would be in standing. At the same time, lift your left knee up, with your knee bent. Your left thigh should be parallel to the floor. Allow the rest of your left leg to hang naturally, with the toes pointing slightly upward. Simultaneous to raising your left knee, raise your left hand in an arc

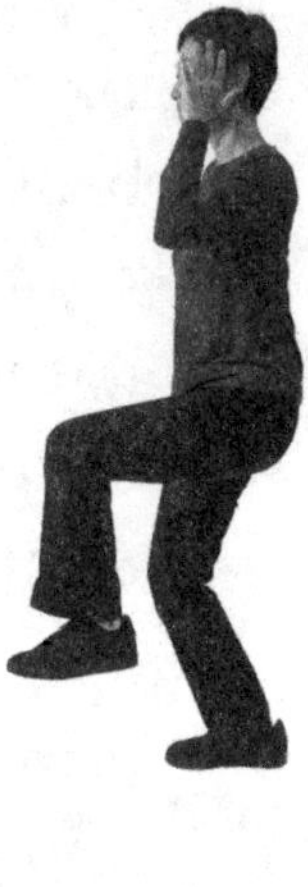

with the elbow bent, as if saluting. The palm should face the side of your check. Stop when your left hand is beside your face. Your right hand should hang beside the hip joint, fingers pointed downward, palm facing your hip. Look straight ahead.

3. Return to a half-squatting position by placing your left foot down, while your right leg moves behind you and your left leg is slightly forward. Your weight is now on your left leg (full). Lower your left hand in an arc and stop when it is beside your thigh. The palm should still face inward. You are now in the opposite stance shown in the photo in the first instruction above.
4. Now straighten your left leg to a standing position and lift your right foot off the floor while bending your knee. Again, your right thigh should be parallel to the floor with the lower half of your leg hanging down. Your right foot is even with the ground. As you make these adjustments, bring your right hand up in an arc and allow it to rest with the palm toward your face.

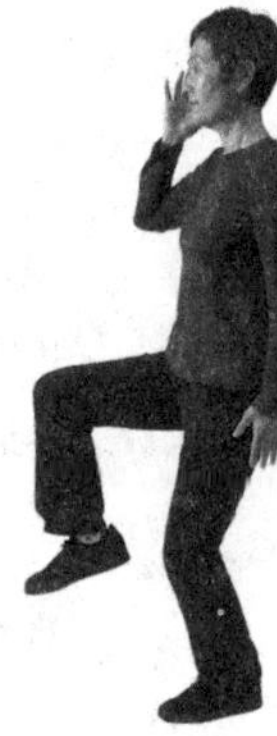

Lower your right hand in an arc and rest that arm beside your hip, fingers pointing to the floor.

5. Continue these moves for the duration of the walk.
6. After completing the Golden Rooster Walk session, stand in the Wu Ji position (described in Step 7 of the Cat Walk) for a minute longer to center yourself and clear your mind.

The Bear Spirit Walk

In many cultures, the bear symbolizes power, strength, and protection, though it can also reflect a sense of calm and wisdom when it hibernates. When doing the Bear Spirit Walk, you effectively alternate between these feelings of power and calm.

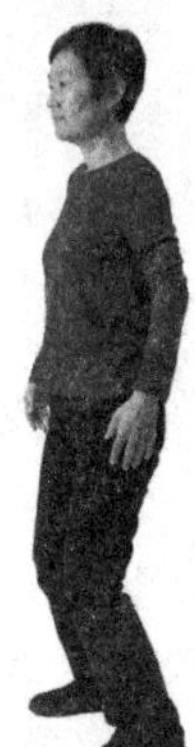

1. Begin by standing with your feet wide apart and your arms raised up to be level with your hips.

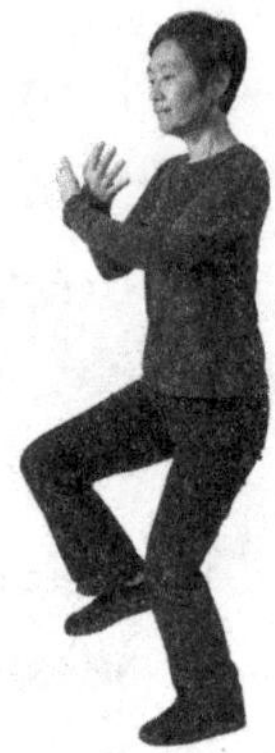

2. Step forward with your left foot, and raise your right leg while crossing your arms. Your right hand needs to be on the inside nearest your chest, palms facing upward.
3. Then take one step forward with your right foot, uncross your arms and spread your hands outward, palms facing down, with rounded shoulders and upper back like a bear.

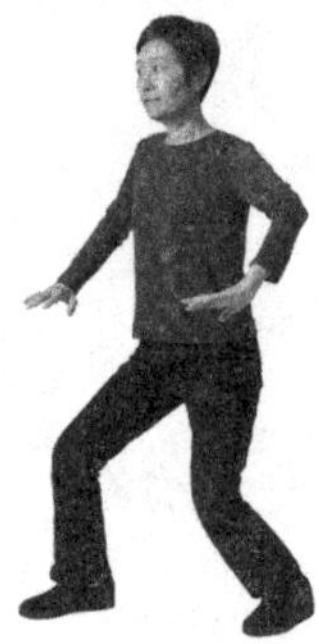

4. Then step forward with your right foot, raise your left leg and cross your arms once again in front of you. Your left hand needs to be on the inside, closest to your chest.
5. Then step forward with your left leg, uncross your arms again, and raise your right leg.

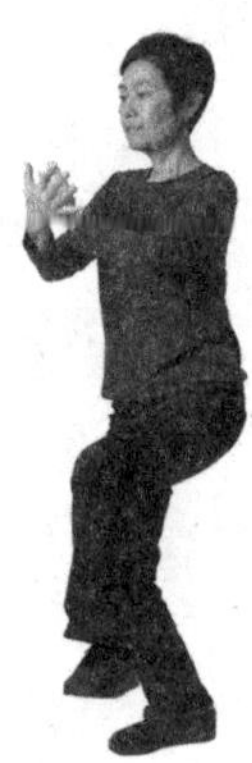

6. Repeat these alternating stepping moves as if you are walking like a bear. Step forward with one leg, cross your arms, and raise the other leg. Then step forward with that leg while uncrossing your

arms, then raise the other leg and cross your arms again.

Tip for Learning the Animal Walks

Be patient with yourself as you learn the Tai Chi Animal Walks. As you begin, proceed at your own pace and give yourself the necessary time to learn the movements.

Furthering Your Tai Chi Study

Once you become comfortable with the three Tai Chi Animal Walks described in this chapter, you may decide that you'd like to further explore this graceful internal martial arts form. In many cities throughout the world, tai chi classes can be found. A Yang-style short form is often taught, including between twenty and forty movements, so it is easy to begin a practice and develop yourself. Classes are often taught at local YMCAs, adult education centers, community colleges, senior centers, and Veterans Administration facilities.

The Continuing Evolution of Tai Chi

The practice of tai chi is no longer just for martial arts devotees. Tai chi has truly become mainstream, and its ranks of practitioners will continue to grow, so we hope you will join in and practice it in a park near you.

Tai chi, with dedicated practice, can become a soothing, calming exercise you can do any time you feel stress building in your daily life. The benefits of tai chi for your overall health are numerous, particularly in helping you build a strong awareness of your inner body's systems. With passage of time, you will find yourself maintaining a youthful, graceful movement that belies your years. If you are already an older adult, begin a tai chi routine and you may even regain years of mobility.

WEEK 6

The Circle Walk for Self-Reflection

The Tao moves by returning
In endless cycles.
By yielding, it overcomes,
Creating the ten thousand things . . .

—Dao De Jing

One of the most reassuring patterns in nature is the circle. From the shape of the sun and moon to the roundness of many trees and roots, the circle represents steadfastness, harmony, and completeness. It is therefore not surprising that for centuries ancient civilizations have used a pattern of circular walking as a method of strengthening their spirit and connecting with the energy of nature.

The final walk you will learn in this book—the Circle Walk for Longevity—is based on a circular moving meditation pattern that originated among Daoist hermits. The Daoists believed that a long healthy life was required to achieve their spiritual aims. As a result, they explored many methods to increase their lifespans. One of their discoveries was circular walking practices. In the second century, these practices were adapted into a new martial art called Ba Gua that is highly esteemed throughout the world for its superior maneuverability.

One philosophical root of the Circle Walk is the concept that everything flows in a circular process of birth, death, and renewal. Day flows into night, and night back into day. Spring departs but returns the following year. The planets revolve around the sun time and time again. Even we as human beings live our lives in cycles. Each morning, we wake up refreshed, then expend our energy as the daytime hours pass, then go to sleep, and finally meet the new day renewed again. Finding inner peace within yourself is also an essential theme of the Circle Walks. This walking meditation provides the vehicle that can transport us to our inner peaceful realms.

It's not certain when circular walking practices began. One reason for the lack of historical records may be that those who practiced it kept themselves in seclusion in the high mountains. As a result, few outsiders knew of their practices. Another reason is that thousands of years of human history and culture were passed down orally rather than in written form. It is therefore impossible to precisely date the circular walking practices or even where they originated.

However, it is likely that the practice of Circle Walking has deep roots, as it can be found in many ancient spiritual traditions throughout history. The Circle Walk was used in ancient China for meditation and as a way to strengthen one's body. Native American tribes performed circular dances around a fire to honor their ancestors, the earth, and their divinities. Prayer circles in which people prayed as they moved around a sacred object were practiced in Judaism, Buddhism, Christianity, and Islam.

The Deeper Significance of the Circle

In many cultural traditions, the circle is a symbol of a deep meaning. In the Judeo-Christian tradition, the circle represents wholeness, eternity, and perfection. Some associated it with God's love for all creatures or God's all-encompassing watchful eye on Earth. The circular halo you see in countless paintings above the head of an angel or saint is said to symbolize sanctity or being connected to heaven.

In Daoist philosophy, the circle is embedded in the hexagon (eight sides) shape, which held an important connotation. The hexagon was often used to determine the best course of action in a difficult situation. If individuals could not decide what action to take, they tossed coins upon a hexagon. The points where the coins landed were then interpreted for meaning. This use still exists today. (In fact, you may see a hexagon above the entrance of houses in Asia.)

In one classic Chinese version of the Circle Walk, the hexagon serves as a type of energy map. As you move around it, you figuratively walk through the universe and encounter eight types of energetic qualities that you need in order to navigate through

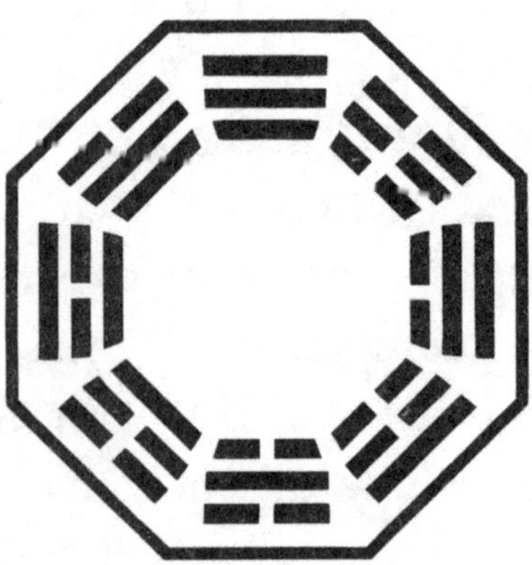

life. The circle that your steps form is thus divided into eight sections, called trigrams, as shown below. Each trigram is coded with lines of various long and short lengths (broken or whole). Each one holds a specific meaning. Going clockwise around the hexagon, here are the meanings

1. Ch'ien (creativity)

This trigram equates to Heaven. Its attribute is strength. Heaven is seen as strong because it moves and never stops. It is the ancestor of all the other energies.

2. K'un (receptiveness)

This trigram evokes an image of the Earth. It is associated with yielding and a quality of gentleness. The earth yields and, as a result, produces many things.

3. Tui (joy)

This trigram represents a Lake. Its attribute is pleasure. Low-lying areas where lakes form are excellent places for spiritual reflection. Power is hidden in the lake's deep currents.

4. Ken (stillness)

This trigram stands for Mountain. It is associated with resting. There is mystery in inner stillness and a sense of a new start. A mountain can withstand a challenge and remain undisturbed.

5. K'an (the deep)

This trigram depicts Water. It is tied to danger. We are reminded to proceed with confidence even in turbulent times in order to achieve success. Water adapts to any circumstance.

6. Chen (arousing)

This trigram denotes Thunder. Its attributes are movement and vibration. Thunder calls us to action with sudden energy and explosiveness. This energy vibrates.

7. Li (clinging)

This trigram stands for Fire. It is associated with brilliance or light. Fire clings to whatever it contacts, transforming its host.

8. Sun (gentleness)

This trigram stands for Wind. The wind can penetrate any opening and travels great distances. Its power is unseen and unpredictable.

As you learn the Circle Walks in this chapter, you might wish to meditate on the qualities of these trigrams to see if any of them hold personal meaning for you. Even if they don't, you can take your inspiration from the fact that the circular nature of the walks deeply imitates the many cycles of life, such as the seasons of the year, the time of day, birth and death, and so on.

Yin and Yang in the Center of the Circle

The yin/yang symbol is often placed in the center of the energy hexagon, as shown in the illustration.

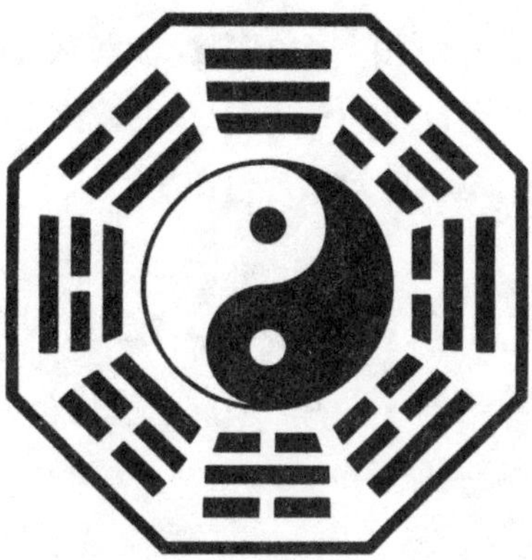

This traditional Chinese symbol represents how the opposing, yet harmonious energies remain in balance. Yin/yang energies can be interpreted as those related to the polar opposites of heaven/earth and internal/external. Other yin/yang pairs are cold/hot, dark/light, night/day, and rest/activity. We learn to live in harmony with the universe only by understanding and accepting the interdependency of the paired elements of nature.

Yin and yang energies exist within each of us. However, the ratio of these energies fluctuates over time. What's important is to project the level of energy that's best suited to each particular situation. One must thus be open to changing energies, if necessary. These two principles apply to all of life. As you do the Circle Walks, the shifting of energies equates to the shift from non–weight bearing to weight bearing, rest to action, and breathing in to breathing out. Such changes are best handled by moving with the flow rather than with resistance.

Health Benefits of the Circle Walks

The Circle Walks offer many health and longevity benefits. Here are some.

Conditioning of the Upper and Lower Body

It is important to engage in physical activity so that you will be able to maintain your physical condition with the passage of time. Circle Walks are an enjoyable and effective way to keep up the strength in your legs. Like the Tai Chi Animal Walks, the Circle Walks gently exercise the joints and major muscle groups of the lower body. During the walks, the knees are bent, and the body is slightly lowered. This builds the muscles of the hips and legs more efficiently than if the legs were straight (as in regular walking).

Meanwhile, holding the arms in a specific static position as you do in the Dragon Walk—which we will teach you shortly—engages the muscles of the upper body. This helps you train and strengthen both the major and secondary muscle groups and tendons, which in turn enable you to better hold your upper body in place during your everyday activities.

The walks also directly increase the conditioning of the torso area. Through the repeated change of direction, the torso area (spine, waist, hips, pelvis, and inner thighs) is made stronger and more flexible.

Increased Body Awareness

The two Circle Walks are the most demanding of the exercises taught in this book. As you will see, walking in a straight line with the inside foot and a curved line with the outside foot requires concentration. At the same time, you must maintain a particular upper-body posture during the walk. The walks also cause you to orchestrate your entire body movement and think of yourself as one unit. Like the Tai Chi Animal Walks, you are training your body to maintain balance during the periodic shifts in direction. All these requirements add up to an improvement in body awareness.

Increased body awareness is important for all of us, but it is especially important for older adults. Numerous studies have shown the risk of falling rises at a startling rate after the age of fifty. A fall that breaks a hip or leg bone can cause a short-term loss of mobility as well as other problems. Worse, not being able to walk often leads to a downward spiral in health. If you maintain a high level of body awareness, you are more likely to notice when you are using your body improperly throughout the day. Thus, you can make adjustments.

Lymphatic System Massage

The importance of the lymphatic system to our health is well established. One of the functions of this system is to help recycle fluids and other materials used by various parts of the body. The lymphatic system also assists in distributing antibodies and white blood cells throughout the body and is thus an integral part of the immune system. During the walks, the lymph glands in the pelvic and inguinal area receive a gentle massage, especially during the changes of direction. Thus, the walks help flush and circulate this area of waste products.

Cardiovascular Health

Many research studies prove that physical activity does not need to be vigorous to provide cardiovascular benefits. The Circle Walks are an effective form of low-intensity, cardiopulmonary exercise. The heart is not as overstressed.

Immune System Functioning

We know that regular physical activity delivers benefits to the hormonal glands and brain centers involved with the immune system. With some other forms of exercise, you risk injury and possible reoccurring physical problems. In contrast, the walks in this book produce benefits with much less impact on the joints and thus a much lower risk of harming a body part or system. Among the immune system–related gains that have been found from practicing the various walks in this book, including the Circle Walks, are an increase in lymphocytes, improved T cell function, reduced production of cortisol, and an increase in the production of endorphins.

Benefits from the Meditative Quality of the Walks

The Circle Walks are often used as a form of meditation, under certain belief that a moving meditation is more powerful than a stationary one. A moving meditation enables the practitioners to develop a keen awareness of their energy center in a way that can be carried over to the movements of everyday life.

The Circle Walking meditation also trains the body to retain "rootedness in motion." In bending your knees and lowering your center of gravity (as well as lowering your Dan Tian, the area below the navel; the qi area), you are better able to gain a sense of stability while performing the circular walking. The shifts in direction as you walk also train your body and mind to stay centered during change.

Meditating while in a standing position alters the experience of centering oneself. There is a higher sense of alertness than with a sitting or reclining meditation. The Circle Walks were designed to enhance inner energy while opening practitioners up to the energy of nature and the universe. The result is a harmonizing of the many energies available.

Stress is reduced during Circle Walking practice. As we pointed out in chapter 1, walking and other physical activities increase the level of endorphins and neuropeptides in the brain. Higher levels of endorphins (which include enkephalins, beta-endorphin, and dynorphin) and neuropeptides (such as dopamine) elevate mood and create a sense of calm and well-being. In addition, the increased oxygen supply in the brain due to walking and breath work improves thought clarity, memory, and concentration. Combined, all of these physiological factors help to create a sense of well-being, which further helps you relax your entire body. Given that a high percentage of illnesses are stress related, adopting meditative practices like the Circle Walks can be an effective self-treatment.

Studies of meditators also have found that they appear to age more slowly. They report better overall physical health, mental well-being, and energy. They have been found to become tired less quickly and sleep more deeply.

Principles of the Circle Walking Practice

In doing the Circle Walks, you will be stepping around an imaginary circle and periodically changing direction. The following are key principles that will help you get the most out of the walks as a type of moving meditation.

Let Go of Physical and Mental Tightness

Remain relaxed throughout the walk. Tightness and difficult emotions held in your body will only make it more difficult for you to enter a meditative state. Scan your body as you move and seek to let go of any tension that you find. If you cannot release the tension, then allow it to remain without adding a layer of judgment about it.

You also want to let go on a psychological level, quieting your mind as much as you can to help prepare yourself for entering a meditative state. If your thoughts are insistent, try counting your steps. You will be surprised how quickly your mind clears.

Breathing exercises will also help release tensions held in your body and help you clear your mind. When your body is not busy holding in all that tension, you have more energy for doing this walk.

When your body and mind are both free of tension, a joyful feeling will surface as you move about the circle.

Find a Slow but Rhythmic Pace

Walk slowly at a steady pace for some time so that you can perfect the footwork. Move at a pace that is slow enough for you to feel comfortable as you step, but fast enough that a natural rhythm emerges. This rhythm will assist in calming your mind. Over time, you will gradually move faster.

Location and Time for Circle Walking

Traditionally, Circle Walks have been performed outdoors to enable the practitioner to absorb the energy of the natural environment. The two walks described in this chapter can be done in your backyard, a park, or some other open outdoor area, but this is not essential. Whether your Circle Walking is indoors or outside, make sure that your path is unobstructed. Give yourself the room you need to move around. Pick a location that is also relatively quiet so you can center yourself during the meditation.

In many places in the world, the walks are done in groups around trees in city parks. In park after park in Asia, you can find the worn paths resulting from the many Circle Walks of practitioners over the years. You can do your Circle Walking around trees if you like. Begin with a circle about five feet in diameter (eight steps). If you do choose to use a tree as your circle's center, select the advanced method described later for switching directions.

The traditional time to perform a Circle Walk is around sunrise or early mornings, because of the clean air and low light at that time. If mornings are not practical for you, choose a time when you will not feel rushed and can enjoy the exercise.

Move with Knees Bent

When you walk regularly, you keep your legs fairly straight, but this is not the case with Circle Walks. Bending your knees helps stabilize your spine and strengthen your legs. This positioning of the legs is often called "sitting thighs." At first, you may want to imagine yourself leaning against a tall stool in order to get the proper positioning.

Use Abdominal Breathing

While you do the Circle Walks, you want to have natural, relaxed abdominal breathing, such as we discussed in previous chapters. If you are still having trouble distinguishing abdominal from chest breathing, do the following exercise, preferably breathing through the nose. First, breathe in a shallow manner in and out of your chest. Next, try to breathe more deeply and allow the air to flow gently down into your abdomen. Exhale. Lastly, breathe in a relaxed manner and visualize the air being pulled smoothly all the way down to the bottom of your torso. Exhale in a relaxed manner as well.

In chapter 4 on the Immune Power Walk, you learned the practice called breathing for healing and energy. Doing breathwork of this type (without any walking) will help you develop proper breathing for the walking practices as well as for everyday use.

Habits to Avoid in Your Circle Walk Practice

Certain habits can work against the smooth flow of movement during the Circle Walks. The following four points cover the most common tendencies by those who are just starting a Circle Walk practice.

Forcing the Moves

You want to maintain a continuous flow of movement without tensing your body in an attempt to push yourself into the next position. Think of it as "going with the flow." A common tendency is making one part of the body rigid in order to build power. This works against using the total energy of the whole body.

Holding Your Breath while Exercising

Have you ever caught yourself stopping your breathing as you try to perform some sort of physical activity?

But holding your breath is counterproductive. Regular, relaxed breathing helps support the movement of your body and enhances the energy flow to the various body parts. Stopping your breath is also a sign of tensing up. Stay aware of your breathing as you do the walks and make sure that it remains smooth and natural. If you catch yourself holding your breath, exhale and start the breathing cycle over again.

Protruding Your Chest

Some practitioners of the Circle Walk protrude their chest and pull in their abdomen as they try to stay balanced during the walks. Protruding the chest blocks qi energy and prevents it from traveling to the Dan Tian area of the abdomen. This can lead to a less powerful energy flow through the entire body. You want to maintain the natural alignment of your upper body. Protruding your chest will make your stances less stable, so avoid doing this.

Bobbing Up and Down

As you perform the Circle Walk, you want to maintain a level height from the floor. At first, you may feel yourself bobbing up and down. Instead, your knees should be bent about the same amount with each step you take.

Preparing for the Circle Walks

You may wish to do some warm-up exercise to stretch and then to center yourself and get into a meditative mood. Here are two short practices:

Standing Like a Tree (Wu Ji position)

1. Stand as still as you can, feet shoulder-width apart. Relax your body.
2. Gaze out in front of you with a soft focus. Look straight ahead, but do not focus on a particular object.
3. Pull in your chin gently and elongate your neck, as if someone is gently lifting you from the top of your head.
4. Bend your knees slightly. During the stance, make sure they do not fall into a locked position.
5. Allow your arms to relax and hang loosely along the sides of your body. There should be some room between your arms and your sides, as if there is a golf ball in each armpit. Your hands should be relaxed as well.
6. Make sure your spine is properly aligned and that neither your stomach nor your behind is sticking out. Both your belly and your hips should be relaxed.

7. Imagine you are being raised from the crown of your head like a marionette. Feel the sensation of elongation that results from your spinal column. Your chest should lower slightly. Relax your shoulders.
8. Scan your body for any area of tension or pain. Depending on your physical characteristics and disposition, you might feel tension in your shoulders or neck, between your shoulder blades, or in your lower back or hips. Release the tension from different parts of your body. As for pain, you might feel a slight burning sensation in your leg muscles due to the slight knee bend, but let it reside there for as long as you can until you have achieved your goal. This pain will decrease with each practice.
9. Inhale and exhale in a relaxed manner through your nose. Continue to relax. If you have thoughts, let them come and go naturally.

This is a traditional position that is compared to standing like a tree. As you do this stance, picture an image of stillness in your unconscious mind. Seek to be at peace with the earth, like a tree in winter, patient and accepting.

Basic Circle Walk: The Tiger Walk

When you are ready, you can start the basic Circle Walk, often called the Tiger Walk, because it imitates the image of a tiger and its spirit. The tiger position connects you to the earth with your palms facing the ground, holding a small ball.

As you do the Tiger Walk, it is important to have an awareness of where the center of your circle is. This is considered the most important location of the circle. On a symbolic level, the center point represents your energy center or the Dan Tian (located about four finger widths below your navel). When you first begin walking, sense the location of both your circle's center point and your Dan Tian as you take your steps. This helps you retain a sense of stability as you move about the circle. You may even wish to place a small object at the center point of your circle to help you keep an awareness of it. Once you feel comfortable with the advanced method of switching directions, you can use a small tree as your center point.

The stepping method you will be using is called the "mud-walking step," also known as the "gliding step." This is one of the most common stepping methods in Circle Walks and is often used to train beginners. This step is helpful in maintaining balance and stability.

You'll want to take the same number of steps around the circle each time. We recommend starting with sixteen steps, and then with practice, move down to twelve and then eight. Assuming an average sized stride, sixteen-step circle will be about ten feet wide, a twelve-step circle about seven and a half feet, and an eight-step circle about five feet. Once you have traced a complete circle in one direction five to ten times, switch and travel in the opposite direction. (We'll use five turns around the circle in the rest of this explanation.)

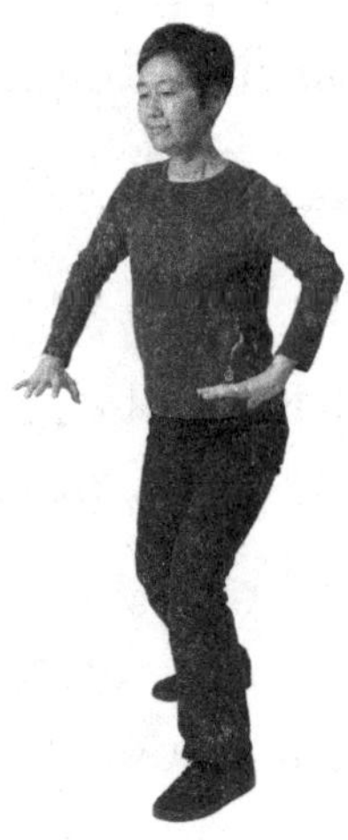

1. Stand at the twelve o'clock position on your circle and face yourself to travel counterclockwise. (Your left side will be inside the circle.) Your right foot should be slightly ahead of your left foot. Bend your knees slightly,

as if you were resting your buttocks against a tall stool. Place your hands slightly away from your body to either side. Your palms are facing down. Leave room under your arms, as if there were a golf ball in each armpit. Your shoulders should be relaxed.

2. Remember that as you make your way around the circle, the positioning of your upper body will remain stationary; only your lower body is engaged in movement. Don't forget to keep breathing into your abdomen. Raise your left foot slightly off the ground, no more than about an inch or so. As the foot moves forward, it should remain flat and parallel to the ground. Step forward in a smooth and consistent manner. Keep in mind that you are stepping as though you are walking through mud.

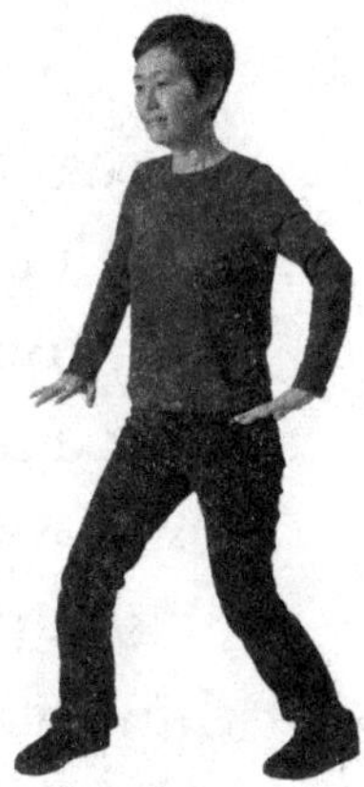

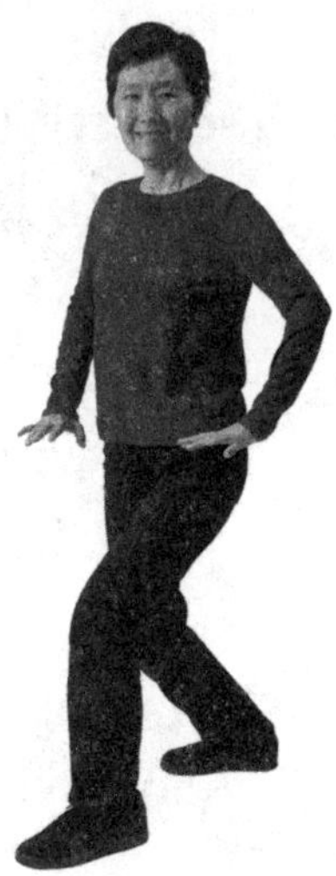

3. Place your left foot down so the entire bottom of your foot hits the ground at the same

time. Your left foot should now be ahead of your right foot.

4. Move your right foot ahead in the same manner as you did your left foot. The only difference will be that your right foot will land at a 45-degree inward-facing angle. This will enable you to end up with a circular path. Remember that your foot should be raised no more than about an inch off the ground.
5. Continue to step around the circle in this way, with your inside left foot landing straight and your outside right foot landing at a 45-degree angle. When you are about to reach the twelve o'clock position for the fifth time, it is time to think about switching directions. When you are using the yin/yang (basic) switch, continue to the six o'clock position before changing directions. If you are using the advanced method, you should switch when your left foot is in front around the one o'clock position when proceeding counterclockwise. Execute the switch using one of these methods. (Both switching methods are detailed below in the next section of the chapter.)
6. Having switched directions, continue clockwise for five rotations. If you are using

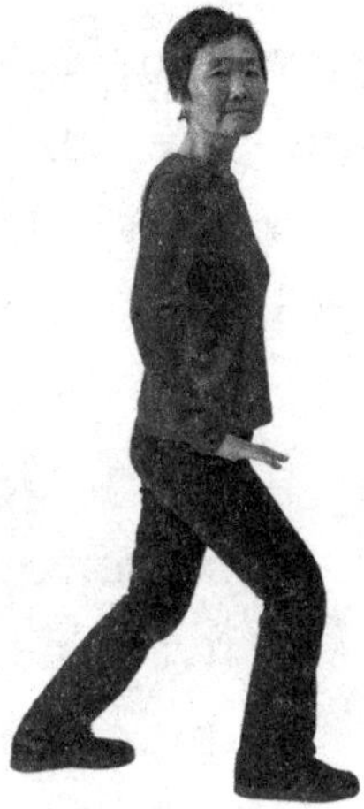

the basic switch, continue to the six o'clock position before switching. If you are using the advanced switch, make the change in direction when your right foot is at the eleven o'clock position.

7. Continue back and forth around the circle for the desired length of time.
8. After you feel at ease with the change of direction, you can do it at any point on the circle.

Traditionally, one Circle Walk consists of three hundred trips around the loop. However, this is a lot for a beginner, so we suggest you begin with about ten minutes of practice. Build up with an additional sequence of five loops in at least one direction each time you do the walk. Eventually, you can do the walk for as long as a half hour to an hour.

Learning the Two Switching Methods

As you just read, you want to switch directions once you have returned to the twelve o'clock position on your imaginary circle after five times around. Here are instructions for two switching methods.

Yin/Yang Method

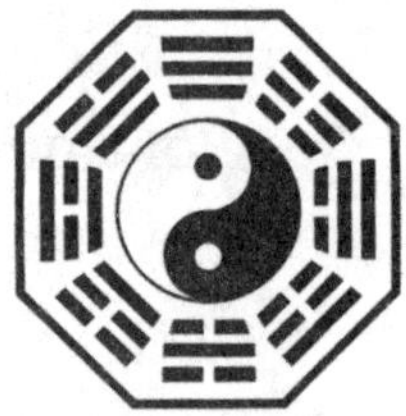

1. Once you have traced the circle five times in a counterclockwise direction, continue stepping until you reach the six o'clock position. As you approach the position, begin picturing the yin/yang symbol in your mind.
2. Turn into the circle and step along an imaginary S-shaped line that separates yin from yang. You will end up back at the twelve o'clock position but heading in the opposite direction. Now proceed around the circle in a clockwise direction.
3. Walk around the circle clockwise for five circuits. Pass the twelve o'clock position for the fifth time and continue now to the six o'clock position. This time, picture the S of the yin/yang figure facing the opposite direction.
4. Turn into the circle and step along the imaginary S line until you reach the twelve

o'clock position. Proceed around the circle in a counterclockwise direction.

5. Apply this switching method whenever appropriate during your Circle Walk.

The Advanced Switch

In the advanced approach, you will accomplish the change in direction by using a series of steps that will actually turn your body around at about the same place you started on the circle. Here are the specific directions:

1. Once you are about to complete five trips around the circle in a counterclockwise direction, start thinking about changing direction around the two o'clock position. You will actually make the switch at around the one o'clock position when your left leg is in front.
2. With your left foot ahead, bring your right foot forward and turn it so that the toes of your right foot meet the toes of your left foot at a 45-degree angle. Your right foot will be facing toward the circle. Your feet will form a V, similar to a snowplow or the braking position your feet are in when you are skiing downhill. In Ba Gua, this is known as the Kuo Bu position.

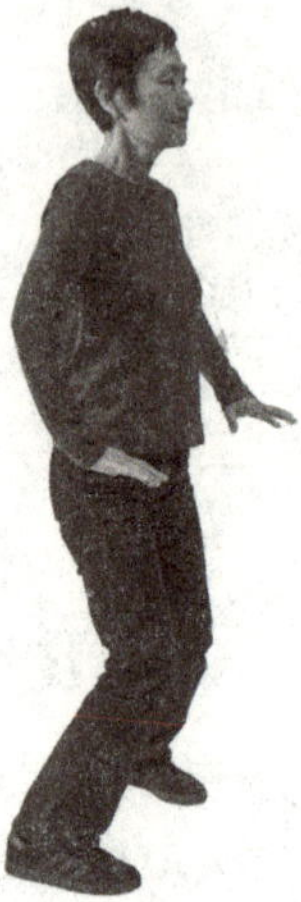

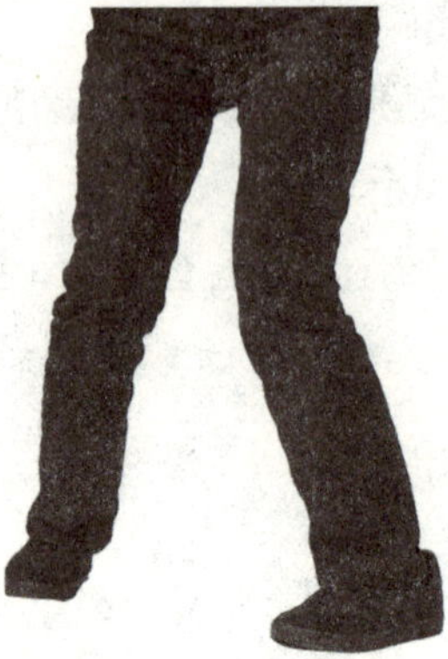

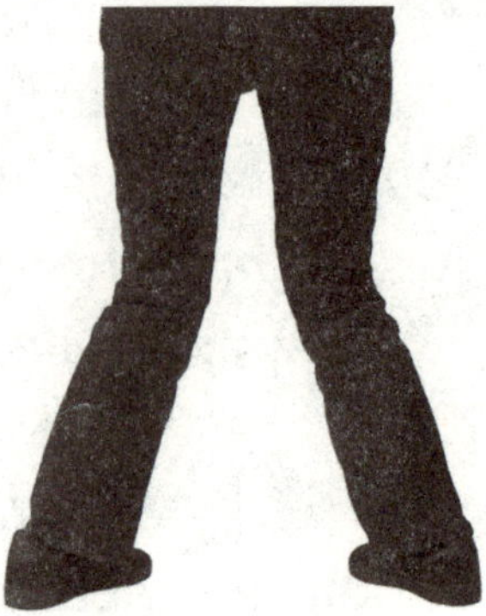

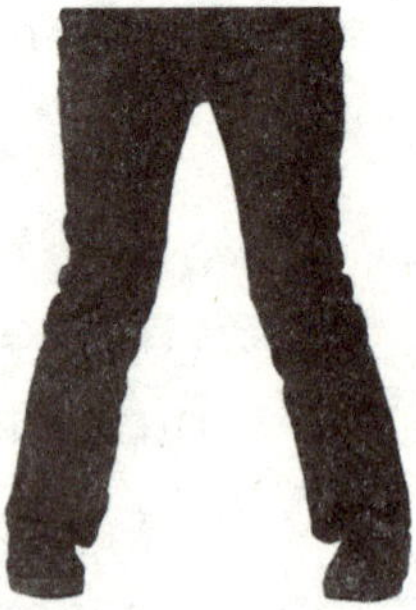

3. Now move your left foot and turn it so it is parallel to your right foot, but with the toes facing the opposite direction. In Ba Gua, this is called the Bai Bu position.
4. To continue the turn, bring your right foot forward again and turn it to form another V (as you did above). Your right foot is headed toward the bottom of your circle. Your feet are again in the Kuo Bu position.

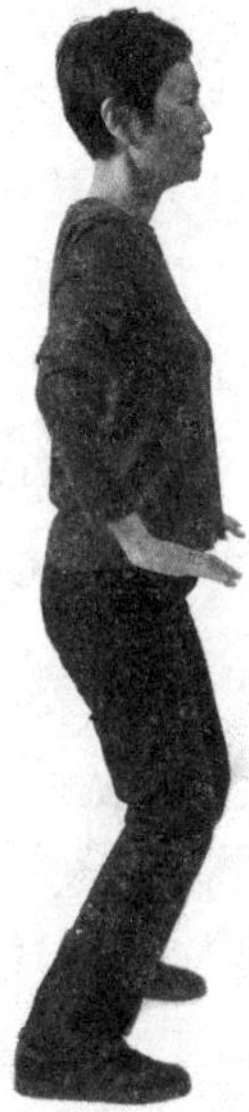

5. Now complete the turn so both feet are back in the mud-stepping position, moving your left foot so it is parallel to your right foot. You have now switched directions and will be walking clockwise.
6. Proceed in this clockwise direction. When you are about to complete your fifth rotation, start thinking about making the directional change when you get to the ten o'clock position. You will actually make the change at the eleven o'clock position when your right foot is forward. (See the diagram on page 169.)

7. With your right foot ahead, bring your left foot forward and turn it so the toes of your left foot meet the toes of the right at a 45-degree angle. Your left foot will be facing toward the circle, and your feet will form a V.
8. Now move your right foot and turn it so it is parallel to your left. You will be facing into the circle.
9. To continue the turn, bring your left foot forward again and turn it so you form another V. Your left foot will be facing the bottom of the circle.
10. Now complete the turn. Both feet will be headed toward the bottom of the circle.
11. You are now positioned to proceed in a counterclockwise direction.
12. Continue your circle and apply the advanced switching method when needed.

Walk the Circle

This diagram shows how to switch directions from clockwise to counterclockwise. Think about making the switch as you are approaching eleven o'clock. When your right foot is in position R2, turn your left foot so that it faces your right foot, as shown in

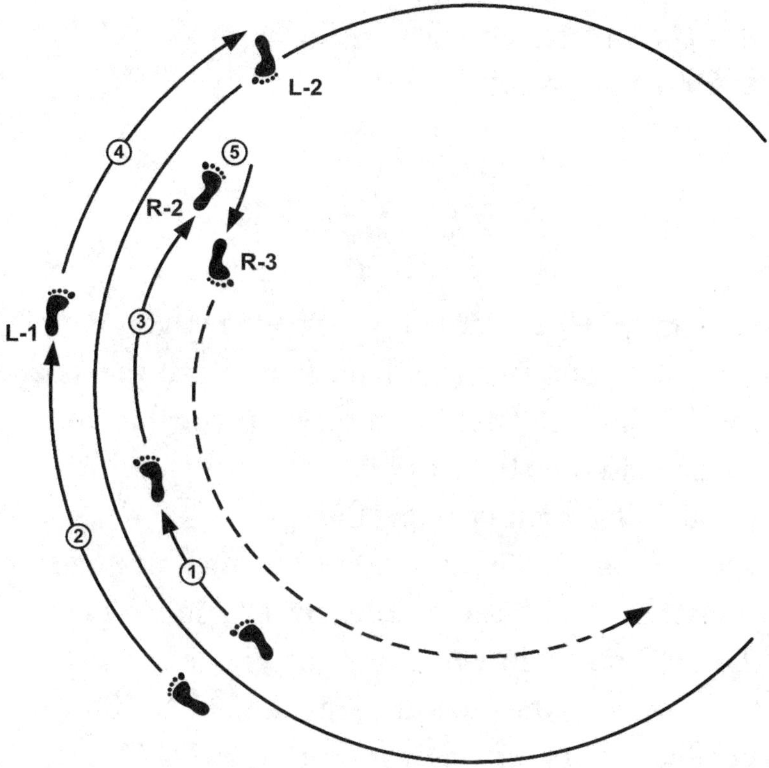

L2. This is the Kuo Bu position. Next turn your right foot, so that it is facing counterclockwise, as shown in R3. This is the Bai Bu position. Switching from counterclockwise to clockwise is the exact opposite of this diagram, in the one o'clock position, with your right foot on the outside of the circle.

The Advanced Circle Walk: The Dragon Walk

The advanced Circle Walk is called the Dragon Walk because it symbolizes a dragon flying into the sky. The walker's position is like a tiger, except that your arms are held out slightly below shoulder level with your palms facing up toward the sky.

Masters of this walk sometimes offer dramatic demonstrations of their skills by moving quickly in the Dragon Walk while holding glasses of water in the palms of their hands, with no spills. (If you would like to try this as you perfect your Dragon Walk technique, we suggest you use plastic cups first.)

The Advanced Circle Walk—The Dragon Walk

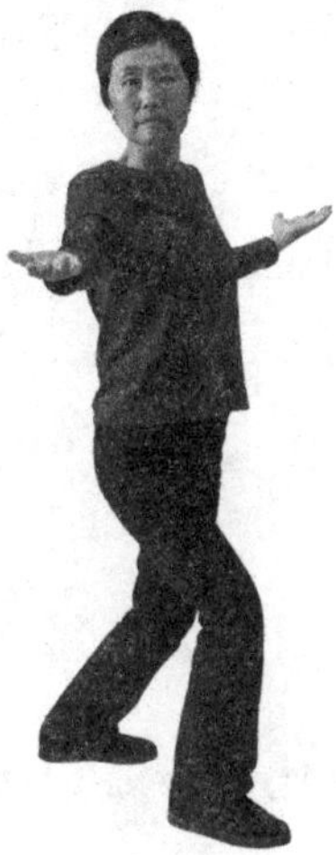

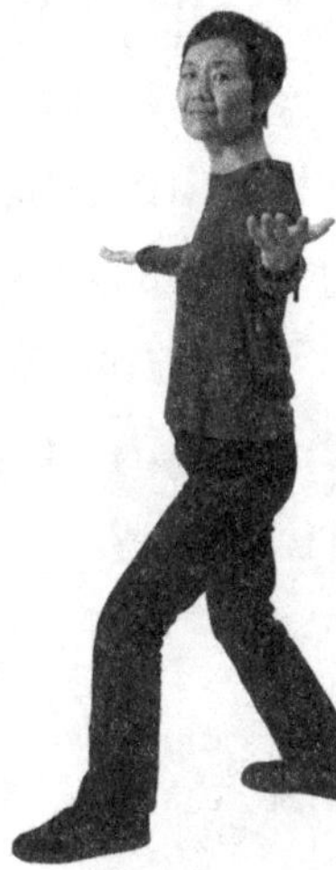

Another view of the Dragon Walk arm position, showing the left side to the circle's center.

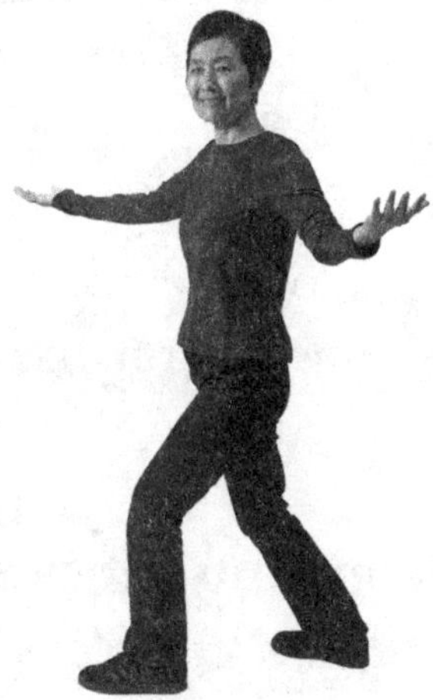

Another view of the Dragon Walk arm position.

Making Circle Walking an Everyday Practice

The Circle Walks do not have to be a formal practice, reserved for when you are ready to exercise in a meditative frame of mind. You can use these walks in a casual way when you are at airports, subway stations, or anywhere where there's room to move around. Place your hands in your pockets and proceed to

Circle Walk in a relaxed manner to pass the time. If you don't have pockets, simply allow your arms to hang at your sides. You can work on perfecting your footwork during this extra time that's become available to you. If you feel uncomfortable using either the basic or advanced switching methods in public, try walking in a figure eight when you want to change directions or simply turn in a way that's easy for you.

Congratulations

You have completed all the chapters in this book that cover the types of walking styles you can add to your traditional daily walk or do independently. These walking styles can revitalize your general health, add years to your life, help you recover from illness, and allow you to become spiritually at peace with yourself and connected to the universe. You have learned about some of the most beautiful exercise practices the human body can perform, all based on simple, yet profound standing or walking positions. As you practice the walking styles in these chapters, may you reflect on these instructions from our esteemed teacher Sun Shurong:

"Cultivate stillness within movement, and movement within stillness—walking becomes a living meditation."

WEEK 7
Integrating the Walks and Staying Motivated

Walk as if you are kissing the earth with your feet.

—Thich Nhat Hanh

There are so many other ways to use walking as exercise. We therefore hope your eyes have been opened to the many different styles of walking you can do beyond the traditional "one foot in front of the other" walk. In our view, it is exciting and fun to try out the various walking styles and mix them into your daily walk. To refresh your memory, here's a quick review of the six walking styles you learned in this book.

Week 1: The Traditional Walk

Of course, you don't need a lengthy reminder about the traditional walk, but let's repeat a few facts to keep in mind. If you are just starting out to create a daily walking routine, begin with a simple goal of 2,000 to 2,500 steps to begin building up your stamina and a passion for walking. Then over a period of a few weeks, try to increase your daily goal incrementally up to about 4,000 steps, then 5,000, and eventually up to 7,000 or 8,000 if possible, according to your stamina and comfort in walking for longer distances. Or think of your daily walks in terms of time, where you aim to walk the recommended 150 minutes per week, roughly thirty minutes a day for five days. But it is also important to listen to your body. You may feel absolutely super one day, with lots of energy and stamina. You would thus have no problem spending time walking long enough to reach 5,000 or 8,000 steps. But on another day, you might feel tired or have pain in your foot or leg. Pay attention to these signals indicating that your walk should be shorter, perhaps just fifteen or thirty minutes, no matter how far you go or how many steps you take. Review this chapter if you want to remind yourself of the other information it provides about age and walking, how fast to walk, treadmill or outside, and the value (and risks) of walking backward.

Week 2: The Vitality Walk

This walk aims to reenergize your inner vitality, your qi energy, so it can circulate throughout your body and revitalize you. While doing this walk, you don't pay attention to steps or distance walked, nor do you listen to your heartbeat or check your pulse. You simply walk and feel the sensation of energy emanating from inside you for whatever amount of time you are comfortable walking. The Vitality Walk is done at a steady, healthy walking pace, and combines a specific breathing pattern with specific walking steps. Your arms are at your sides, with the Adi Mudra position, and your tongue is curled slightly up. The Vitality Walk generally has you inhale and exhale through your nose, not through your mouth. You learned the Basic Walk, with a five-step breathing pattern: First step: sniff in; second step: sniff in; third step: exhale by sniffing out; fourth and fifth steps: neutral breath position (your lungs are empty, and you are breathing neither in nor out). You also learned the Moderate Level, using an eight-step breathing pattern. Review the chapter and video if you need a more detailed refresher.

Week 3: The Mindfulness Walk

This walk is aimed at developing a greater sense of inner peace by helping you focus on psychological rebalancing and spiritual cultivation. Learning this walk involves focusing on being in the moment, quieting the mind, matching your breathing to your steps, and smiling so that you feel joy as you walk. The walk involves specific positions of the hands that aid in achieving a meditative state of mind (the half-a-prayer position) and breathing deeply as you slowly walk and open your senses to the natural world around you. Review the chapter for more reminders of how you achieve the state of mindfulness as you do this walk.

Week 4: Immune Power Walk

This week covered two medical qigong walks that are used to treat chronic conditions caused by a weakened immune system, in particular, as part of the treatment for some types of cancer. The Immune Power Walks are also good as general moderate exercise for anyone seeking to improve their health and to develop flexibility. The walks were created by Guo Lin, a Chinese artist who modified various qigong movements to treat her cancer. The movements and breathing patterns of the qigong walks help calm the nervous system, moderate the heartbeat, lower blood pressure, reduce muscle tension, and deepen breathing. The style of the walk involves a preparatory deep abdominal breathing pattern and during the walk, a special breathing pattern similar to the one for the Vitality Walk along with a coordinated stepping pattern. This walk may take time to become familiar, so review the chapter and the video to ensure you know how to do it.

Week 5: The Tai Chi Animal Walks

In this week, we taught you three practices that involve movements mimicking animals—the Cat Walk, Golden Rooster Walk, and the Bear Spirit Walk—and utilize movements that come from tai chi martial arts movements. By doing these walks, you learn to maintain balance while gracefully performing a series of physical moves that alternate between inaction and motion, as you change the way you carry the weight of your body from one leg to the other. The Animal Walks thus promote both strength and agility in the lower muscles and joints. Maintaining leg strength is important for staying fit. The walks are also useful for those with arthritis, osteoporosis, and back pain, as well as to improve cardiovascular conditioning. Review the chapter for the specific instructions on how to do the Cat Walk,

Golden Rooster Walk, and Bear Spirit Walk and watch the videos.

Week 6: Circle Walk

The purpose of this walk is to enter into a meditative mindset. The walk is based on a circular moving meditation that originated among Daoist monks thousands of years ago. In the Circle Walk the knees are bent and the body is slightly lowered, thus gently exercising the joints and major muscle groups of the lower body. The arms are held in a specific static position, thus engaging the muscles of the upper body. This helps you train and strengthen both the major and secondary muscle groups and tendons, which in turn enable you to better hold your upper body in place during your everyday activities. During this exercise, you walk around an imagined circle or an actual physical object such as a tree, periodically changing direction using a specific foot pattern. You use natural, relaxed abdominal breathing. The basic Circle Walk is called the Tiger Walk, as you are imitating the slow, intentional movements of the tiger as it circles its prey. The advanced walk is called the Dragon Walk because it represents a dragon flying into the sky. Review the chapter for the many benefits you will obtain in doing this walk and for the specific instructions on performing each one.

Suggestions for Incorporating the Walks into Your Daily Traditional Walk

As we said earlier in the book, you can integrate many of the other walking styles into your traditional daily walk. Alternatively, you can choose some of the various walking styles and use it as your entire walk for the day, performing it for thirty minutes to an hour. Here are some suggestions for ways to combine the walking styles:

Combinations with the Traditional Walk—One-Hour Walks

Here are some ways you can combine the walks taught in the book. In general, it is best to begin with the easiest walk as your warm-up, then switch to a different, more strenuous walk.

1. Start with your traditional walk for twenty minutes, switch to the Vitality Walk for twenty minutes, then finish with the Mindfulness Walk for twenty minutes.
2. Start with the Vitality Walk for forty minutes and finish with the Immune Power Walk for twenty minutes.
3. Start with a slow traditional walk for twenty minutes, switch to the Japanese walk

for twenty minutes, then finish with the Mindfulness Walk for twenty minutes.

4. Start with the Mindfulness Walk for twenty minutes and then continue with the Immune Power Walk for twenty minutes and finish with Vitality Walk for twenty minutes.
5. Use any three walks of your choosing for twenty minutes each, or select two walks and do them for thirty minutes each.

Combination of the Animal Walks

1. Start with the Cat Walk for ten minutes, switch to the Golden Rooster for ten minutes, then end with the Bear Spirit Walk for ten minutes.
2. Start with Cat Walk for ten minutes, Golden Rooster for ten minutes, and continue with Tiger Circle Walk for ten minutes.
3. Start with Bear Spirit Walk for ten minutes, Tiger Circle Walk for ten minutes, and Dragon Circle Walk for ten minutes.
4. Any three combination practices from Cat, Golden Rooster, Bear Spirit, Tiger Circle, and Dragon Circle.

One Walking Style per Day

Some days, you may not have as much time or you may simply feel less motivated to do a thirty-minute or an hour-long walk. So, assess your needs and just get started with a short walk that appeals to you. Are you feeling especially stressed? Go outside and do one of the Circle Walks for as long as you like. Would you like to develop more body awareness? Try one of the Tai Chi Animal Walks. Would you like to have more energy? Switch to the Vitality Walk. Would you like to be more balanced and centered? Try the Mindfulness Walk. The variety of walks described will help you stay motivated and on track.

How to Sustain Your Motivation to Walk

We hope you are now excited to begin integrating all you have learned in this book into a regular walking routine. But the key question is: can you stay motivated to go for a walk at least five days per week or even every day?

It comes down to being and staying motivated. Of course, motivation is an individual matter. Each of us is motivated by different things and we choose our goals in different ways. To get motivated, we each need to find the key to our own ignition. To help you, we have five reasons for you that might help you decide what motivates you the most. As you review the following explanations for increasing your drive, you'll hopefully feel that one of them speaks more directly to you than others. That is a good sign, as it is probably because it relates to an area of your life that you most strongly, perhaps unconsciously, want to improve. So read these reasons with an open mind and see which ones powerfully call out to you.

Reason #1: Achieve Overall Better Health

Hippocrates is credited with saying, "Walking is a person's best medicine." Walking helps you achieve gains in your overall health no matter what your age or gender. Right away, you'll start to feel less stressed, have more physical energy, and enjoy more restful sleep. Even better, the long-term health benefits from a regular program of even moderate daily walking are vast and impressive. Many studies have shown that walking helps prevent chronic diseases, aches and pains, and the process of aging.

Here is a quick reminder of the many benefits you can derive from walking on a regular basis:

- Lowers your risk of heart disease
- Strengthens the heart by increasing blood circulation to heart tissue

- Promotes better circulation throughout the entire body
- Lowers blood pressure
- Reduces the risk of cancer
- Lowers the likelihood of developing type 2 diabetes
- Reduces the risk of osteoporosis
- Walking strengthens muscles and aids in joint stabilization
- Improves lung capacity
- Helps manage your weight
- Tones muscles, improves the mobility of our joints, and helps prevent loss of bone mass and bone fractures
- Helps mitigate overeating
- Assists in stress relief
- Improves thought clarity, memory, and concentration
- Helps you age more slowly

The more consistent you are in taking regular walks and integrating the walking styles presented in this book into your daily walk, the more of these benefits you will obtain. The best way to make this happen is to begin thinking of walking not as exercise but simply as one of your natural daily activities.

Reason #2: Improve Your Emotional Well-Being

Once you become involved in a regular walking practice, the emotional benefits become apparent very quickly. A daily walk can give you a new perspective on whatever concerns you are pondering and is a release for stress and pent-up tensions. You will also feel a sense of pride because you are taking the time to care for yourself. The calming aspects of the walking practices in this book add another dimension—training you to remain centered in the midst of any turmoil.

Another emotional benefit of exercise is a type of natural "high" that comes from the mood-elevating hormones in the body—particularly the endorphins in the brain—that naturally increase during physical activity. The high you get from walking is also a result of becoming involved in a rhythmic activity that creates a sense of being in harmony with the passing of time. Feelings of calmness while working out come from taking in more oxygen and having less carbon dioxide in the bloodstream. The higher oxygen supply clears your mind and sharpens your thinking.

Studies have found that the emotional benefits from a walking program are cumulative. Over time, the self-esteem and self-confidence of the regular exerciser rise. Studies also show that exercise is beneficial for conditions such as anxiety and depression. One meta-study published in the *British Journal of Sports Medicine* even found that physical activity is one and a half times more effective at reducing mild-to-moderate symptoms of depression, psychological stress, and anxiety than medication or cognitive behavioral therapy.[1]

Reason #3: Getting More Years of Enjoyment Out of Life

A number of studies indicate that many of the declines associated with aging are simply the result of a lack of physical activity. Without physical activity, the body's systems deteriorate. Muscles lose strength, the body becomes stiff and less flexible, the heart and circulatory system weaken, and cognition declines.

Studies have shown that exercise is vital for healthy aging. Along with a healthy diet, those who exercise have more energy and motivation to live a fuller life. They suffer from fewer aches and pains and, due to physical activity, they have fewer chronic conditions. Physical activity helps people reduce anxiety and stress as well as sleep better. A general state of good health allows you to continue to engage in sports, travel, and other activities. In short, it goes without saying that the better you feel as you age and the fewer health problems you have, the more you can enjoy all that life has to offer.

Reason #4: Boosting Your Longevity

Throughout this book, you have read about the longevity benefits of the various walking routines taught. These exercises give your whole body a tune-up. The various systems of your body—circulatory, muscular, skeletal, respiratory, immune, digestive, lymphatic, and so on—all receive benefits.

Regular walking, even as little as two hours per week, also helps prevent a key change in DNA—the shortening of telomeres, which are the protective caps at the ends of chromosomes. As we explained in chapter 1, in the normal process of cell division, the telomeres get shorter over the years. Eventually, if they become too short, the ends of the chromosomes can fray or stick to each other. Telomere shortening is thought to be an element in causing cell multiplication to go askew (which can lead to cancer) as well as an accelerator to aging. Walking, however, can prevent telomere shortening or even lengthen them. In an analysis of over 400,000 British adults from the UK

Biobank, researchers found that people who walk at a brisk pace can be as much as sixteen years younger in terms of biological age versus their chronological age by the time they reach midlife.[2]

Reason #5: Getting Financial Savings

Staying in shape physically, emotionally, and mentally will literally save you money over your lifetime. First of all, you'll most likely avoid many unnecessary medical expenses, including prescription drugs, doctor visits, and hospitalizations. As you plan for retirement, you will have fewer concerns about how you will pay for medical expenses in addition to your other needs. Of course, you'll still need to be properly insured and prepared but your total medical expenses in your twilight years are very likely to cost less.

Consider some hard figures about your risks and costs. As we mentioned earlier, those who do not engage in physical activity regularly are more prone to a range of chronic health problems. More than 150 million Americans have a chronic condition. Specifically, six out of ten Americans suffer from one chronic condition, while four out of ten suffer from two or more. About 30 million Americans have five chronic diseases. While the costs of treating chronic conditions are often paid for by insurance companies or a government program such as Medicare, many people must pay a portion of those costs (co-payments and/or deductibles), and those without insurance must pay all the costs.

So why not improve your chances of avoiding the costs associated with chronic conditions? Engaging in physical activity today is like putting money in a savings account for the rest of your life. You will have a reserve that you can draw upon during times of emergencies.

Seven Practical Tips to Boost Your Commitment

In addition to the five reasons to stay motivated, we also want to provide you with some practical tips you can use on a day-to-day basis for supporting your commitment to walking. Keep in mind that part of continuing to engage in a daily walking regimen is making it as accessible and appealing as possible. These suggestions can help you with new ideas to keep up your motivation.

Tip #1: Feel a Sense of Pride

Be proud of yourself and realize that by committing yourself to a routine of being physically active, you've taken responsibility for your own health. You are trying walking styles and movements that are probably very different from anything you've ever done. By exploring physical activities that are new and stimulating, you've eliminated the boredom factor that can creep into the traditional "one foot in front of the other" walking style. Now you've become acquainted with a perspective on movement that is likely new to you, one that inspires you to expand your attitudes toward fitness and health.

If you open yourself up to new ideas about your body and how it moves, you will begin to develop a new attitude toward exercise. You don't need to believe that strenuous physical activities are the only means you have to achieve health. Instead, there is an entire world of other types of exercise and movement that can help you reinvigorate your muscles, your mind, and your spirit.

Tip #2: Reward Yourself

Periodically consider giving yourself a reward for staying on track. It could be a visit to the spa, a professional massage, or a trip to a beautiful location where you can walk in nature. It's smart to support the progress you've already made with some type of positive reinforcement. Note that rewarding yourself doesn't have to involve an item or activity that goes against the healthier way you are conducting your life. There are many ways of acknowledging yourself that are supportive of your new choices. But once in a while, it's okay to indulge yourself with a treat.

Tip #3: Consider Finding a Walking Partner or Starting a Walking Group

Many people are motivated when they pair up with another exerciser to help keep their exercise commitment. Two or more people can support each other and hold each other accountable. Note, however, that this is not true for everyone. Sometimes it is more convenient to go by yourself; no need to wait for another person. A study at the University of Florida found that women who worked out alone did better. The researchers concluded that the convenience of solo exercise was a major factor. In the study, about fifty women between the ages of forty and sixty were instructed to walk for thirty minutes five times a week. Half the group walked alone, whereas the others traveled to a certain meeting point and strolled from there. Over a period of fifteen months, the solo exercisers were more consistent with their walks. They were also more likely to continue to the end of the study. In weighing your options, consider your personality, schedule, and lifestyle. Some people enjoy the social aspect of exercise and would benefit from enlisting an exercise partner.

Tip #4: Rotate Your Walking Locations

One way to keep your exercise routine fresh and fun is to have a variety of locations where you walk. Think about the various parks in your area and choose those with different ambiences. One may be lakeside, another in the woods, and a third on a mountaintop with views of the city or surrounding hills. When you work out at home, pick various spots around the house or in the yard. If the weather's bad and you feel comfortable performing the practice, walk at your local mall. Weekends are a good time to travel to locations that are farther away. No matter where you walk, be sure to have some water on hand. Also, pick locations where you'll feel safe and remember to always stay alert.

Tip #5: Use Positive Self-Talk to Deal with Internal Resistance

Some days it's harder to get yourself moving than others. If you find yourself resisting doing your walking regimen, start to listen to the negative self-talk that's going on in your head. For every reason your mind produces for not exercising, come up with a convincing argument for working out. For example, if you tell yourself, "I really need to work late," try a response like "I'll be more productive if I leave now to take a walking break." If the negative message is "I'm really too tired to walk today," come back with "I'll burn off stress and feel more energetic if I exercise."

You can also create your own supportive messages or affirmations—short phrases you silently repeat in your mind or write down on notecards. An affirmation states your intended result as if the development were already true. It should be a real possibility that reflects a positive change in your life. The following are some suggested affirmations that will assist you in staying motivated and committed to your new exercise regimen:

- Every day and in every way, I am healthier and healthier.
- I have time for exercise, and I will find it.
- Fun and easy, fun and easy.
- Growing stronger and healthier every day, learning a lot along the way.
- One hundred days, one hundred blessings.

Feel free to create your own affirmations. Keep them short and rhythmic. Use rhymes if you can think of them. If you find yourself resisting a particular message, try a different wording or thought.

Tip #6: Take Advantage of "Found Time"

We all have those days when we unexpectedly have free time on our hands. Maybe an appointment was canceled, or the car's in for service and you're stuck at home. Perhaps a project you were working on at your job took less time than you anticipated.

Make the most of the situation. Reread the chapter covering the walking practice you most enjoy, and check your movements against the instructions in the book. Or start to learn another of the walks. Then take some time and go to a park you've never been to before. Instead of staring at your device for hours, motivate yourself to make progress with your exercise program.

If you find that it's becoming more difficult to do your workouts, look at practical ways to make it easier. Just setting out your exercise clothes and shoes the night before may give you that extra push you need to get moving the next morning. Would having another set or two of workout clothes help? If so, make a point of purchasing new ones so there are some clean clothes to grab when you're rushing to get to your workout.

Tip #7: Start an Exercise Journal or Diary

A diary or journal can be helpful in many ways. First of all, you can use it to plot out your exercise schedule. Looking at your plans one week at a time, you can see whether there are any conflicts coming up that might interfere with your practice. Will you need to change the time on a particular day because of a conflict with work or family obligations? You can also jot down the time you actually do put in each day, along with any specific progress, insights, or difficulties you had. Was there an obstacle that made it hard to work out? How can you prevent this from occurring in the future? Are you giving yourself enough time to relax and enjoy the workout? Perhaps you need to leave the office or set the alarm for fifteen or thirty minutes earlier.

Be sure to note the specific practices and warm-ups you do as well. In addition, write down any inspiring thoughts or ideas you have about your exercise program. Whether you're on a routine of your own design or using one of the plans we've described, the exercise diary will provide a visual record of your progress. You can occasionally scan the pages to see what conditions serve you best and what gets in your way.

Another value of an exercise diary is to keep track of how exercise helps you discover more about yourself and perhaps develop higher levels of awareness. Cultivating a high state of awareness during physical activity can lead to deeper self-knowledge. Rather than listening to music or a podcast, try staying in tune with your body and the sensations you are feeling during the walking and movement exercises in this book and write your experience down in your journal after the activity. The meditative walks can be particularly valuable in inspiring new insights into yourself. In this way, you discover how to accept yourself, without judgment. This higher level of self-awareness then carries over to your daily world where you start becoming aware of habitual behaviors and reactions that do not serve your best interests. This knowledge is the first step to developing healthier and more productive ways of being as you mature and age.

Walking: Exercise for a Lifetime

We are confident that the versatility and proven effectiveness of the exercises in this book make them perfect lifetime companions for you. Each walk in this book is unique, so you can switch from one to another as your needs change or as you simply wish for more variety in your life. If you already have an exercise routine, the walks and exercises in this book can be used in combination with whatever else you are doing—swimming, bicycling, hiking, and so on. Keep moving in the years ahead and enjoy your walking!

> *When the mind moves, the qi moves; when the qi moves, the body follows—walking thus becomes a flow of spirit and form.*
>
> —Sun Shurong

APPENDICES

APPENDIX A
Nutritional Guide for Health and Longevity

Now that you are taking better care of yourself by beginning a walking program, we would like to offer you some basic guidance about nutrition and a healthful diet. We use the word *diet* to refer to the many types of food you eat during the day, not to the meaning of dieting wherein you punish yourself and try to eat less food. Diet in the sense we use it in this chapter is a neutral word, one that simply means all the types of food you eat.

Learning how to eat for better health has become increasingly important to people of all ages in the industrialized countries of the world. There is a growing recognition that having good health and avoiding disease are highly correlated with one's diet. For example, nutritional research has revealed how a diet high in carbohydrates (rice, pasta, bread, bakery goods, pizza, etc.) is linked to obesity, high blood sugar, and type 2 diabetes. Other research has linked ultra-processed foods with increased risks of cancer, cardiovascular disease, obesity, type 2 diabetes, and premature death. On the other hand, research suggests that eating carbohydrates with a low glycemic index (e.g., low in glucose) can lead to lower blood sugar levels and that carbohydrates with high fiber content are beneficial for digestion and the immune system. Ultimately, there is no shortage of research to support the linkage between many types of foods and good health versus chronic conditions versus life-shortening diseases.

There are scores of books devoted to proper nutrition and eating for health, and this brief chapter cannot go into the depth of information you will find in them. However, we would like to support your new walking routines with basic information on how to construct a diet and eating habits that support your vitality, energy, and overall good health. We believe that the goal of eating is not just to feed your body, but to nourish it. What you eat and how you eat need to build your muscles, provide your cells with the wide range of nutrients that supply their energy, and keep your immune system healthy to prevent illness.

Nutritious foods also power your brain and help you manage stress, a key contributing factor associated with many diseases.

Eating the right amount of food is also important to avoid weight gain, especially as you age. Avoiding overeating combined with a regular walking routine can help you lose unwanted weight if you need to, or at least maintain a healthy weight. With regular walking, it is likely that you will see excess weight naturally drop off over time. If you walk just five hours a week at a moderate speed, you can lose about a pound in two weeks without dieting (in this use of "dieting," we do mean restricting your food intake). However, we do not emphasize weight loss in this chapter and discourage you from following any strict self-regulating food intake methods such as calorie counting. Instead, we offer guidance for understanding the fundamentals of how to make the best food choices.

The Four Principles of a Healthy Approach to Food

In the past decades, numerous books have appeared proposing their unique program of foods to eat and be healthy. You may recall these programs: the South Beach Diet, the Beverly Hills Diet, the keto diet, the

Mediterranean diet, the Asian diet, the Japanese diet, the cabbage diet, the raw food diet, and many others. We do not endorse any one of these specific programs as they are, in general, too restrictive for most people to consistently follow. Rigid food regimens don't work very well given human psychology. Most people find it hard to abandon foods they grew up with and they prefer to eat whatever attracts them in the moment.

What we recommend instead is a program of eating based on four general principles of nutrition. These principles reflect a mixture of what we would consider the best cuisines that, in our opinion, support eating for nutrition and good health. These cuisines are the Asian diets, the Mediterranean diet, and the keto diet. These diets generally emphasize eating a wide range of vegetables, fruit, and healthy proteins such as fish and chicken, along with fats from oils and nuts. While some of these cuisines allow for the consumption of grains, others do not. They generally include less red meat and no processed foods. Moreover, our version of healthy eating allows for personal taste when it comes to creating your meals.

In our recommendation, the four foundational principles are: simplicity, moderation, temperance, and seasonal eating. Here is an explanation of each one.

Simplicity

A simple diet focuses on eating vegetables and grains, with smaller amounts of the other types of foods. There is little emphasis on beef or pork, but alternative sources of protein, such as fish and soy foods, are used amply. Fruits are enjoyed in season. This way of eating is quite different from the Standard American Diet (SAD) that contains an unhealthy amount of meat, sugar, and fat, as well as many artificial foods (margarine, synthetic sweeteners, nondairy creamers) and an array of processed foods loaded with chemical additives. Americans typically do not eat enough fresh vegetables and fruit, which are vital to a healthy diet that prevents most chronic conditions. Many research studies show that individuals who overindulge in food and do not exercise suffer more health problems than the active people with simpler diets.

Today, Western fast-food restaurants serving fat- and carbohydrate-loaded convenience foods are spreading throughout Europe, South America, the Middle East and Asia. We are now seeing young children and teens in many countries who have obesity problems, and some with type 2 diabetes, both of which were previously rare in those cultures.

Moderation

This principle is self-evident: overindulging in food can lead to weight gain, obesity, and a plethora of chronic conditions such as type 2 diabetes, cardiovascular disease, and the following five physical disorders:

- Frequent defecation
- Frequent urination
- Sleep disturbances
- A body too heavy for exercise
- Indigestion from taking in more than can be absorbed

Learning to eat in moderation can be difficult for people who love food, but it can be done. It involves reconnecting with the body's signals of hunger and satiation. If you are tempted to eat every few hours all day long, you are likely not listening closely to your body's real signals of hunger. Practice paying attention to the body while eating and try tasting the food and enjoying the sweetness, saltiness, or pungency of each bite, instead of being on your device or thinking about what you will do after the meal. Further, it is important to chew your food thoroughly so that the food mixes with the digestive enzymes in the saliva. Intentionally slowing down the eating process, chewing well, and savoring each bite of food can help you become more attuned to your body's signals to stop eating.

Making a commitment to eat with moderation can take time, because it requires developing a greater awareness of your body's messages. At first, you may just need to become familiar with how it feels not to eat to fullness rather than overeating. Most people are at least familiar with what their stomach feels like when they've overstuffed it with food (like on Thanksgiving). So, begin to tune in to how much food you're eating and how full you feel. In a short time, you'll become aware of how much food it takes to feel full. Eventually you want to aim for about 80 percent of that feeling of fullness at mealtime.

Experiments have shown that a regular practice of undereating brings health benefits and increases lifespan. A lower-volume diet lowers blood sugar and cholesterol, keeps liver enzymes at youthful levels, and supports the immune system. Restricting your food intake results in greater alertness, less likelihood of heart and kidney disease or cancer, and a higher overall feeling of well-being. In contrast, overindulgence, especially with nonnutritious foods, leads to congestion, indigestion, depletion, and deterioration.

Temperance

Temperance is the third key principle in a healthy approach to eating, which means having some self-restraint. Instead of using common sense, people sometimes veer to extremes in their food choices and eating habits. They may begin eating a particular food too often because it has been the focus of recent health news, but in doing so, they are actually being counterproductive to good health. An example of this is the trend toward drinking "smoothies" every day. Blended fruit drinks provide far more fruit sugar than a real piece of fruit.

Temperance also includes unnecessary self-restraint with an occasional indulgence. An infrequent treat should not be considered a reason for guilt and self-reproach. Instead, you should be gentle with yourself. In fact, giving yourself a little leeway can help you stick to a healthier overall diet.

When you have an attitude of temperance toward your diet, your behavior changes. You are in a better emotional space to sensibly work on having your nutritional needs met on a regular basis, knowing that an occasional splurge is fine. You can begin to make smarter choices that produce ongoing feelings of natural energy and well-being.

Seasonal Eating

As our fourth principle, we suggest that a major key to eating for nutrition and longevity is to focus on eating foods locally grown in the season you are living in. Seasonal eating not only helps you live in harmony with nature by priming the body to cope with the changing environment around you, but also ensures you are consuming the freshest foods whose nutritional values (like vitamins, minerals, and proteins) are at their highest.

Many traditional cuisines around the world have long emphasized seasonal eating (largely because they had to be based on using local ingredients before global trade made foods from around the world available to them). The delicious dishes of Mediterranean cooking always utilize the freshest vegetables, fish, and meats of the season.

Ancient Chinese culture is perhaps the most deeply linked to seasonal eating. The Chinese concept that the universe contains two polar opposites —yin and yang—applies not just to philosophy but also to food. Some foods are considered to be yin, meaning they have a cooling and calming effect. Yin foods are thus eaten in spring and summer. Yang foods are considered to be warming and stimulating and are eaten in fall and winter. Some foods have an equal amount of yin and yang, and are called balanced foods. Some examples of the three types of foods are:

- Yin foods (cooling): tropical fruits, salad greens, milk, sugar, honey, and yogurt
- Yang foods (warming): root vegetables, potatoes, barley/oats, eggs, butter, cheese, and meat
- Balanced foods: many local vegetables, beans, seeds, nuts, fish, and many whole grains (including brown rice)

If you follow this classification of foods, you would not eat a hamburger for lunch in summer, as it will increase the heat in your body. Similarly, you would benefit from a beef and root vegetable stew in winter to warm up your core.

Today, with the wide availability of refrigeration and long-distance shipping of foods from around the world, it is far easier to eat a wide variety of foods in any season. In some cases, it can also be healthier, such as having fresh oranges from Chile in winter if you live in Wisconsin, or fresh fish from the Atlantic Ocean if you live in Oklahoma. Nevertheless, try eating seasonally and see if the foods taste better and help you feel healthier.

Your Body's Need for Protein

When it comes to protein, the principle of moderation is key: neither too much nor too little. In the US, large portions of meat have long played a starring role on our dinner plates, while vegetables, potatoes, and so on were only supporting players. Americans still tend to overconsume meat by about one and a half to two times the daily levels recommended by the US government. Trendy high-protein weight-loss diets only encourage this tendency. Meanwhile, some vegetarians in this country underestimate their need for protein.

The problem is, recommendations for protein consumption vary widely, depending on the individual. The US Recommended Daily Allowance (RDA) for protein is 0.8 grams a day for every two pounds of body weight for adults. This translates into about 46 grams of protein for an average-size woman and 56 grams a day for an average size man. If you are small or large framed, you need to make an adjustment. However, be aware that the World Health Organization gives a much lower recommendation of 35 grams a day.

Here's one way to determine your own protein needs. Just three ounces of chicken breast—about the size of a deck of cards—provide about half of your protein requirements for the day. In US measurements, you only need a total of five to seven ounces of protein per day, and some of this will come from other food sources.

Here's a review of the various sources of protein you have.

Red Meat (Beef)

The Chinese and Mediterranean diets do not use much red meat in their cooking. Agreeing with this principle, we encourage you to minimize your intake of red meat or even to eliminate it from your nutritional program. Except for very expensive cuts of red meat, much of it has a high-fat/high-calorie content and has been treated with hormones and antibiotics. On occasion, if you want red meat, try to purchase organic beef.

Eating red meat tends to cause you to overdo your protein intake. The following examples show

how much protein is in just a small three-ounce serving of different types of beef:

- Lean bottom-round roast beef: 26.9 grams
- Extra-lean ground beef: 21.6 grams
- Rib eye steak: 23.8 grams
- Sirloin steak: 25.8 grams
- Filet mignon: 24 grams

Considering these amounts, you can see how easy it is to exceed your daily requirement if you are eating the usual large cut of beef (10- to 16-ounce) typically served in restaurants or purchased in supermarkets.

Other Meats

Chicken is a staple meat in most countries around the world. Many styles of cooking make excellent use of small pieces of chicken in stews and stir-fries, such as with soy sauce and ginger for seasoning. Chicken is healthier if the skin is removed. The breast is the leanest part of the chicken, containing less than half the fat of a T-bone steak. A three-ounce serving of chicken breast (without the skin) offers 26.7 grams of protein. Choosing naturally raised (organic) chicken is a way to avoid residual hormones and antibiotics.

Some people believe that pork is an unhealthy meat to consume, but in the past decades, the pork industry has improved the methods used to raise pigs for consumption. Pork is high in protein, B vitamins, and essential minerals such as zinc and iron. However, choose lean cuts of pork such as tenderloin, loin chops, and sirloin roast, as other cuts can be high in cholesterol and fats.

Lamb is often an overlooked choice on many people's menus, though sheep are the most numerous livestock in the world. This type of meat is consumed in many cultures in Central and East Asia. The foreshank is lower in fat than other cuts and is the best choice. A three-ounce serving of foreshank lamb contains 26.4 grams of protein. Lamb is rich in infection-fighting zinc and also has potassium and magnesium. It provides carnitine, which is needed to metabolize fat in the body.

Other Sources of Protein

You can also obtain protein from many alternative sources in addition to meat. Consider these alternatives:

Fish

An excellent source of protein, fish is known to cause a lower incidence of heart disease. Research has shown that fish oils have a positive influence on creating a healthy balance of high-density lipoproteins (HDLs, or good cholesterol), low-density lipoproteins (LDLs, or bad cholesterol), total cholesterol, and homocysteine (a type of amino acid). Fish is also easier to digest than meat, low in saturated fat, loaded with vitamins and minerals, and a source of all the essential amino acids.

Most supermarkets today offer a wide assortment of fresh fish, although much of it is now farm raised rather than our preference for wild caught. Salmon is a good choice, as a small 3.5-ounce portion provides 27 grams of protein. Canned sardines are another nutritious choice because they are rich in protein. One two-ounce can contains about 12 grams of protein.

When buying fresh fish, keep the following tips in mind. The scent of fresh fish is light and sealike. It should not smell strong or "fishy." Check to see whether the eyes are bulging, clear, and shiny—or sunken, cloudy, and opaque. The first description is characteristic of fresh fish.

Tofu

Also called soybean curd, tofu is a rich source of protein that is lower in fat and more easily digested than meat. Made from soybeans, water, and a curdling agent, its neutral taste gives tofu the ability to absorb the flavors of whatever it is cooked with. Tofu becomes an even better source of protein when it is combined with brown rice, such as in a tofu burger or stir-fry dish served with rice.

Tofu also contains phytoestrogens, natural substances that can provide benefits to people in midlife. Phytoestrogens (found in good quantities in soybeans, soy milk, and tempeh as well) have been shown to help reduce the symptoms of perimenopause (the symptomatic years before menopause) and menopause in women. Men are finding tofu and other soy-based products useful in their efforts to reduce enlarged prostate glands.

Tofu comes in four different types—soft, regular, firm, and extra firm. The more firmly tofu is pressed, the more protein it contains. Three ounces of firm tofu (about one-fourth of a block) contain 6 grams of protein; the same amount of extra firm has 10 grams or more. Be sure to check the expiration date on the package and select the freshest tofu you can find. A sell-by date of ten days ahead is preferable. Don't buy tofu if the package has bubbles or bulges.

Tempeh

This is a fermented soybean product that can be purchased in Asian markets and health food stores. Tempeh has an even higher protein content than tofu—15.7 grams per half-cup serving. Tempeh is also lower in fat and contains more fiber. It has a meaty texture and can easily replace ground meat in recipes. You'll find tempeh packaged in sandwich-sized squares that can be used to make a quick and easy lunch. Choose the freshest tempeh available at the store.

Miso

Another soy product from Asia, miso is a fermented paste used by the Japanese to add flavor to soups, dressings, stocks, and other foods. You might be familiar with miso soup at Japanese restaurants. Miso is often made of soybeans, salt, and water, but may also contain barley, rice, or chickpeas. Miso becomes darker and more strongly flavored the longer it is fermented. A dark miso has a heavy flavor that enhances hearty soups or stocks. A light miso is sweeter and more delicate tasting, so it is good in salad dressings or less filling soups.

A benefit of consuming miso is that it offers live lactobacillus cultures and digestive enzymes.

Serving-size portions of miso are usually less than half a cup. This small amount provides 16.3 grams of protein.

Eggs

Eggs are a protein-rich food. One hard-boiled egg provides 6.3 grams of protein. However, the research on consuming eggs has been confusing as it seems to change periodically. The most recent verdict, however, is that adults can consume up to seven eggs per week without affecting their heart health. Eggs supply 6 grams of protein and are also an excellent source of vitamins A, D, and B_{12}, as well as choline, a nutrient essential in many metabolic steps. For some people, overconsuming eggs can trigger food allergies, including hives, headaches, and other reactions. Also, there are concerns about cholesterol, though recent research indicates that the cholesterol in eggs does not affect the human body as much as other sources of cholesterol.

Dairy Products

Yogurt is a good protein source. A one-cup serving of the low-fat variety contains 11.9 grams, nonfat has 13 grams, and regular has 7.9 grams. In consuming yogurt, you also get digestive support from the lactobacillus cultures it contains. Yogurt is a common staple among people in many parts of the world, from Europe to West Asia, where many people are said to live beyond one hundred years old.

Eaten in moderation, other milk products such as cottage cheese, cheese, and sour cream can be used as protein sources and to broaden the diet. Purchase the low-fat varieties whenever possible. Be aware, however, that such products have been known to trigger food allergies. A half-cup serving of low-fat or regular cottage cheese delivers about 14 grams of protein. Cheese contains different amounts of protein depending on the type you choose. One ounce of feta has 4 grams; mozzarella, 6.8 grams; provolone, 7.2; Roquefort, 6 grams. A tablespoon of grated Parmesan contains 2.1 grams. Two tablespoons of regular sour cream contain 0.9 grams of protein.

Combining Foods to Create Complementary Proteins

You can also mix many types of foods whose partial protein content is complemented by another type of food to create the full spectrum of amino acids your body needs. Some examples of protein combining are beans and grains; grains and nuts; or vegetables with nuts, seeds, or grains. Such combinations are widely used as a protein source by vegetarians around the world. The possibilities of achieving good-quality combinations are vast, and some mixtures even provide more protein than meat. The main goal in combining various foods is to create a complete protein serving containing a full range of amino acids. Nine of the twenty amino acids that are present in the body need to come from the outside, and proteins are their primary source.

Beans complement whole grains such as brown rice to create a full source of amino acids, which is why rice and beans are a popular combination. You can also try some of the "super grains" such as amaranth, teff, and quinoa in combination with beans. The proportion needed to create a full spectrum of amino acids is usually one part beans to two parts grains. It you are relying on complementary proteins, be sure to vary your plant sources with a range of beans (legumes), whole grains, nuts, seeds, and nut butters.

Here are some other combinations you might try: soy milk/amaranth cereal; raw spinach/pine nuts; pecans/brown rice; brussels sprouts/basmati rice; sweet potato/brown rice; brown rice/pine nuts; summer squash/amaranth; cooked cauliflower/brown rice; peanut butter/multigrain bread; or lentils/basmati rice.

Early theories about food combining insisted that combined foods must be eaten in the same sitting.

However, we now know that the body can take advantage of the various protein sources of amino acids if they are consumed separately throughout the day.

Your Body's Need for Fruits and Vegetables

In addition to protein, the body needs a wide range of the vitamins, minerals, and essential elements found in fruits and vegetables. Here are some recommendations to help you place them at the top of your eating regimen.

Vegetables

In recent years, even the US government has been advocating eating far more vegetables and less meat than is typically found in most American diets. Vegetables are good sources of vitamins A (beta-carotene) and C. Many vegetables also provide vitamin B6, potassium, calcium, magnesium, and selenium. Vegetables also supply fiber and are generally low in fat.

Some ways to increase your intake of these health-stimulating foods include:

- Eating an occasional meatless meal, such as a salad or vegetable soup. You will be fine if you don't eat meat at every meal.

- Increasing the proportions of vegetables used in your recipes.
- Filling your plate with more vegetables and less meat.
- Considering enjoying some vegetables (carrot or celery sticks) as a snack food.

Widen your choice of vegetables if you tend to eat only a limited selection of them. Studies suggest that cruciferous (cabbage family) vegetables help protect against both colon and rectal cancer. These include bok choy, cabbage, mustard greens, sprouts, turnips, brussels sprouts, kohlrabi, cauliflower, and arugula. Cabbage family vegetables are best eaten soon after they are purchased, and leftovers should be eaten within a day.

Fresh and Dried Fruits

In a recent US government survey including ten food categories, Americans were found to have the lowest intake of fruit. Fresh fruit is among the best sources of vitamins and minerals, and they supply phytochemicals that help prevent free radical damage to cells. (Free radicals are unstable molecular mercenaries that attack healthy cells in your body and increase the risk of cancer and heart disease.) In today's global trade world, you can usually obtain a wide variety of fresh fruits in any supermarket.

Another way to include fruit in your diet is to eat dried fruits, such as dried apricots, peaches, apples, figs, raisins, and plums (prunes). They are nutrient dense, a good fiber source, and most often low in fat. When shopping, select dried fruit that is free of defects and has a good color. You could also consider making your own dried fruit using a dehydrator.

Your Body's Need for Water

Water should be considered the most important liquid you consume. It is essential for maintaining the smooth function of your body. Water adjusts your body temperature, removes waste products, and is essential for hydration. As part of digestion, water transports vital nutrients, vitamins, and minerals in a solution so they can move through the intestinal walls into the bloodstream and into your cells.

If you are now exercising regularly, it's important to hydrate your body, drinking water as needed depending on your activity and the climate. Try to avoid sodas altogether and keep your fruit juice intake low.

Drinking water becomes even more important as you age. Dehydration is a major problem for older adults and can even result in death. The risk of dehydration increases because of the kidney's decreased ability to effectively process urine, side effects of medications, and other causes. This problem is more pronounced in the elderly, especially among men. A special note to avoid plastic bottles as much as possible due to microplastics.

Drinking Tea

In Asia, you rarely see people drinking a lot of water, but what you will see is tea being sipped throughout the day. Asians have long recognized that tea consumption brings healthful benefits. Many studies have been conducted around the world to research tea's health-supporting properties, including a possible anticancer effect and the prevention of heart disease. Such health benefits of tea are thought to come from polyphenols that have antioxidant properties. Recently, a *New England Journal of Medicine* article cited research corroborating the anticancer properties of green tea when consumed at levels equivalent to two cups each day.[1]

Today it is easy to find a wide variety of herbal teas in supermarkets and specialty stores. Consider starting your day with a warm mug of peppermint tea and relaxing at the end of the day with a cup of chamomile. Peppermint tea aids digestion and reduces gas. Enjoy different types of fruit teas but avoid drinking excessive amounts of any one tea.

Fat Matters

You are probably already aware of the need to be careful about how much fat you consume. Yet despite all the attention the issue of fat has received in our media, most Americans still eat too much. Meat, of course, is a significant source of fat, especially the saturated kind, in the American diet. Research has found that a high-fat diet is a factor in many chronic health conditions, such as obesity, heart disease, diabetes, and cancer.

On the other hand, you can also go too far and not eat enough fat. A moderate amount of fat in the diet is necessary for good health. One reason is that fat provides a medium in which a number of vitamins, such as A, D, E, and K, dissolve. This allows these vitamins to be carried into the bloodstream and delivered to different parts of the body. Also, fats are the building blocks for brain health.

Two of the best sources of fat are avocado and olive oils, which are high in monounsaturated fatty acids. (Note: fatty acids are basic units of fat molecules.) Avoid oils such as safflower, corn, soybean, and sunflower. Omega-3 fatty acids found in salmon, albacore tuna, sardines, and mackerel also have the thumbs-up and are excellent for brain health.

Other Healthy Foods to Include in Your Diet

Many of the healthiest cuisines also include foods that are known to support good health. Here are some of the best ones to include in your meals:

Garlic: For centuries, garlic has been revered by many cultures throughout the world for its medicinal properties and flavor-enhancing ability. Numerous studies confirm garlic's role in warding off infections and acting as an antifungal. Garlic is also thought to have cardiovascular benefits by lowering cholesterol levels. Garlic is a rich source of selenium, which assists in the body's production of antioxidant enzymes.

You can use natural garlic in your recipes, but you can also find it in the form of deodorized supplements that you can take by mouth, though it is uncertain if they have the same effects. The question seems to be how to prepare the supplements in order to maintain or even to enhance garlic's benefits.

Ginger: Numerous cultures have long appreciated ginger for its support of digestion, stimulation of circulation, and various healing properties. In cooking, it can be used in sauces, soups, stir-fries, and desserts. Ginger makes a great seasoning for fish, rice, vegetables, noodle dishes, and salad dressings. Whenever possible, use fresh ginger rather than ground powder. When purchasing fresh ginger, avoid cracked, dry pieces and look for sections with shiny, smooth skin. Store at room temperature. This spice is also a common ingredient in Chinese and Ayurvedic herbal remedies.

Ginger tea can be made easily by adding a few slices of fresh ginger to hot boiled water and steeping it for six to eight minutes. Remove the slices and, if desired, add a touch of lemon juice or a bit of honey to the tea before drinking.

Seaweed: Packed with nutrients. seaweeds are moving from Asian cultures to wider use in the Western world. Nori, dulse, kelp, and Irish moss are all rich sources of calcium, iron, zinc, and B vitamins. Benefits of consuming seaweed include smoother digestion and a lowering of cholesterol.

Kelp is a commonly used seaweed in the US. A brown seaweed, it is used as a flavoring in Japanese soup stocks. Dried kelp is called "kombu" and is black in color. It's the seaweed we often see wrapped around sushi. Kombu is also made as a tea. Nori is found in many Japanese foods. Interestingly, almost a quarter of all dishes in Japan contain some variety of seaweed.

When considering adding seaweed to your menu at home, be aware that seaweeds are sold in a dry form. They must be soaked in water before cooking. Seaweeds can then be sautéed and served on their own like spinach, added to rice or beans while cooking, or blended into soups. Seaweed is also used in salads.

Foods to Cut from Your Diet

As you develop a stronger awareness of the possible negative side effects of the foods you eat, you'll want to learn what to avoid. Over time, you will come to see that what we take into our bodies truly does affect how we feel on a daily basis as well as our long-term health. Here are some of the more troublesome food types that we recommend you avoid.

Fried Foods: Besides producing fat-laden dishes, frying foods in oils creates free radicals, which are cellular invaders that ravage other cells in their quest to replace missing electrons. Nutrients such as vitamins A and C are also destroyed when foods are fried. Deep-frying is the worst method. A short two-minute sauté in olive oil is preferable, followed by the addition of water and subsequent steam cooking at a lower temperature. Even better cooking methods include steaming, broiling, and baking. Today, you can also purchase air fryers, which fry food with very little oil using extremely hot air.

Research studies are zeroing in on frying's specific health impacts. A study at the University of North Carolina suggests that consumption of the type of fats found in fried foods—trans fatty acids—may be a contributing factor in breast cancer.[2] Other studies have linked trans fatty acids to heart disease, indicating that these acids may be even worse for our hearts than cholesterol.[3]

Highly Processed Foods: These have been widely popularized in many Western cultures. More than six thousand synthetic chemicals are used in US foods, and those include preservatives, flavorings, colorings, flavor enhancers, stabilizers, and thickeners. If you look at food labels, you will also find hydrogenated vegetable oils, white sugar, and white flour. Processed foods also often have too much added salt and sugar.

Many people buy packaged processed foods and fast foods because they think these are more convenient. However, getting into the habit of eating clean just takes a little adjustment, and feeling better in the long run will be worth the effort. You will also find that it's more cost effective to purchase foods in their original form. All that manipulating of foods can have its price—on your future health.

Sodas: Many Western cultures are overconsuming soft drinks. One of the reasons routine soda drinking poses a problem is that most of these drinks contain a large amount of sugar (often in the form of corn syrup) and other worrisome ingredients such as caffeine and phosphoric acid. Regular sodas deliver a hefty amount of sugar—on average, seven teaspoons per day for each person in the US. Also, diet sodas contain questionable sweeteners whose impact on long-term health is uncertain. Sodas often replace more nutritious and natural foods in the diet. Added to all this is the growing suspicion that heavy phosphoric acid consumption depletes mineral deposits, particularly calcium, in our bones. Research findings on this last point have been inconclusive, but the best choice for drinking remains water in its unadulterated natural state.

Caveats on Alcohol and Coffee

Paying attention to your intake of these two beverages deserves a special note. First, excessive alcohol consumption is unwise and unhealthy. Our advice is that it's best to avoid more than an occasional drink of alcohol. Beer quenches thirst, but most beers are full of calories from carbohydrates. Current research suggests that alcohol does not have health benefits as previously reported.

Although the popularity of coffee has exploded in the United States, the health record on coffee is actually rather mixed. Caffeine has been linked off and on to ulcers, heartburn, heart problems, breast cancer, and prostate problems, among other ailments. More firmly established has been the addictive quality of caffeine. The best approach to coffee drinking is a moderate one, keeping your consumption limited. If coffee causes you to experience stomach discomfort, headaches, excessive nervousness, or muscular tremors, consider cutting back by drinking half decaffeinated/half regular coffee or switching to non-caffeine teas.

When to Eat

How should you schedule your meals in conjunction with walking? With the exception of the Vitality Walk which is done before meals, all the walks described in the book can be done before or after meals.

Your state of mind and your environment are also important for supporting the smooth function of your digestive processes. We recommend avoiding eating when you are upset because your body will be off-balance. Western science backs this up with studies that have shown that stress negatively affects digestion. When under stress, your mind perceives a threat and begins a response. The physiological changes that occur are complex, but one aspect of this is that your autonomic nervous system slows down. Blood flows away from the digestive tract to muscles to prepare you to fight or flee, so digestion slows down. Researchers have found that stress is a factor in about 60 percent of all gastrointestinal disorders, problems encountered by at least 20 percent of Americans on a regular basis. Some of you may frequently notice digestive discomfort that results from eating when you are upset or rushed, such as taking lunch hours at your desk.

If you find yourself in a tense state when it is time to eat, take a break and try a simple exercise to relax your body. Go to a quiet place and close your eyes. Breathe gently into your abdomen as you do the following.

1. Starting at your feet, move through your body and intentionally relax each part. Move slowly up your legs, into your torso, through your

arms and hands, into your shoulders, and up your neck to your head.

2. If any part is resistant to relaxing, try exaggerating the tension first and then releasing it. This relaxation practice will help bring your nervous system back to normal.
3. When you're finished and relaxed, go enjoy your meal.

A pleasant environment in which you can take your time and relax is the best place for eating. Be sure to chew your food thoroughly to support digestion and assimilation. Relax as you eat and enjoy the color and texture of your food. Savor the different flavors and aromas. With each bite, think about taking care of yourself and nourishing your body. Make each meal an enjoyable ritual in which you are being good to yourself through nourishment.

Taking Charge of Your Own Nutrition

It would be impossible to cover all the factors involved in a complete nutritional program in a single chapter. We have tried instead to give you a helpful overview of what you should emphasize in your food choices and eating habits. We've stressed especially the basic principles that separate many of the most healthful diets found in the world. We hope you will take our guidelines to heart.

As you begin changing your food choices and eating habits, remember that your diet must be tailored to benefit your body and health needs, so keep in tune with your body's messages. Be moderate in your approach and see what foods work best for you. Many of you should find that the guidance described in this chapter will instill in you a general feeling of well-being, increased energy, and more comfortable digestion. In the long run, we believe it will also support better health and longevity.

Appendix B
Clothing and Equipment

As you begin implementing the routines in this book, especially the Vitality Walk, it is important to make sure that you have good walking wear and gear that enhances and supports your efforts. Not only can equipping yourself appropriately be an enjoyable part of the process, it also helps you avoid discomfort or injury. In addition to acquiring the right clothing and gear, you also need to know how to take proper care of perhaps your most important bit of equipment, your feet.

Walking Shoes

The most important item you should consider purchasing is a good pair of walking shoes, particularly if you begin practicing on a regular basis. In fact, we recommend having two pairs of walking shoes that are slightly different so you can rotate them from day to day.

Feet are often the first area of the body to become sore when you begin a walking program. Wearing a pair of shoes specifically designed for walking can help prevent problems. The biomechanics of walking are particular to the activity, and over the past decades, manufacturers have become increasingly sophisticated in designing shoes for specific sports. You don't want to lace up a pair of jogging sneakers when you intend to go walking. Running and jogging shoes have too much cushioning in the heel, which can actually hinder your walker's stride.

Here are the basic features you want to look for in a walking shoe:

- **Overall fit.** Your foot should feel comfortable in the shoe without tightness in the front or sides. Tightness can lead to blistering. Yet you do not want the shoe to be so loose that your foot slides around. When you are standing, there should be about a thumbnail's space between your toe and the front of the shoe. And there should be enough room in the heel that a pencil could be inserted comfortably.

- **Width in the "toe box."** You should have enough width in the front of the shoe to wiggle your toes. This will enable your toes to spread naturally and comfortably during push-off.
- **Flexible forefoot**. At the moment of lifting your toes off the ground, walkers flex their forefoot more than runners do. Bend the walking shoes you are considering and make sure they are flexible around the area where the ball of your foot will hit the shoe.
- **Arch support.** Look for good arch support at the midsole. This will aid proper movement and prevent soreness. If your arches are flat, some brands design walking shoes with arch boosters.
- **Cushioning in the heel.** As mentioned, walking shoes have less cushioning in the heel than running shoes. Yet a certain amount of cushioning is important in walking shoes because walkers tend to strike down harder on the heel. The shoe is effectively absorbing one and a half times your weight with each step. Look for between a one-half- to three-quarters-inch thickness in the heel of a walking shoe. Your heel should feel stabilized by the shoe.

- **Slight flare in heel construction.** Another element of heel construction is the heel flare. In a walking shoe, you want the heel to be wide and flare out a bit. This provides stability and prevents overpronation or supination. Overpronation occurs when the ankle rolls too far downward and inward with each step, leading to strain on the big toe, which does the push-off. Supination occurs when the foot rolls to its outer edge during a step, placing stress on the foot.
- **Sole that provides traction.** Avoid shoes with smooth soles—they provide no traction. Walking shoes need to have waffle-like bottoms.
- **Sturdy lacing system.** The lacing of the shoe should stabilize your foot and prevent it from rotating in or out. Be sure the laces will stay tied, as you don't want to stop your walk every fifteen minutes to retie your shoes.
- **Lightweight.** A good walking shoe tends to be light, usually weighing less than eleven ounces.
- **Materials.** A combination of leather and mesh on the upper part will allow your foot to breathe during your walk. Stretchable

mesh also helps ensure the shoe conforms to your foot shape, which reduces pressure on sensitive feet with bunions or diabetic neuropathy. Also be sure the outer materials are water repellent and easy to clean and even washable in your washing machine. As for the inside of the shoe, be sure there are no seams in the fabric lining to prevent irritation on your foot.

Shop for walking shoes in the afternoon, because feet tend to swell during the day. You want to have both feet measured, and if one is larger, purchase the bigger size to ensure both feet have enough room. Don't feel rushed when you are trying on shoes; take your time to ensure you are buying the right size. If you are not sure of the fit, try on shoes both a half size smaller and larger. This can help you determine which size feels best. Also, be sure to wear the same type of sock you will be wearing when you walk.

Good walking shoes are an investment. We recommend purchasing the best shoes you can afford from a reputable, well-known brand that specializes in walking shoes. A new pair of walking shoes can last for several years and will prevent you from developing painful and costly foot problems, so a higher investment is likely worthwhile in the long term. Also, it is best to buy the shoes at a store where you can spend time trying them on rather than from the internet, unless you have purchased the exact same shoes before and know that they fit you.

You can find many videos about the elements of a good walking shoe on the internet that explain the bone structure of the foot, pronation, supination, the need for arch support, and so on.

Socks

Along with the increasing sophistication of walking shoes have come advances in high-performance socks. Today's well-designed sports socks are capable of wicking sweat away from your feet, as well as cushioning and supporting them. Socks with wicking ability are made from either a synthetic material (CoolMax, acrylic, Polartec, nylon) or a combination of high-tech fibers or wool. Many have extra padding in the heel or toe, areas where there is more impact when walking. Also, make sure the socks you buy fit snugly around your feet. Extra material and wrinkles in socks can cause blisters. You will probably want to stay away from 100 percent cotton socks, because they hold moisture against your skin when they absorb sweat. Some manufacturers make socks for each sport, so be sure to buy socks for walking. High-performance socks cost more than regular socks.

A Foot Maintenance Guide

Once you develop a regular walking or exercise program, nothing can be more frustrating than having it disrupted by sore feet. Consider these suggestions on how to avoid or deal with the foot problems that most often show up in walkers.

Arch Soreness

After extended walking, some people feel soreness in the arches of their feet. If you are experiencing this problem, look at your shoes and make sure they provide adequate arch support. If your feet tend to roll inward because of a lack of support at the midsole, the tendons in the arches of your feet will become overtired. Arch supports purchased from your local pharmacy or a different pair of walking shoes may eliminate the problem.

Walking on hard surfaces also may be a contributing factor, so choose turf instead of sidewalks or asphalt roads for a while and see if the soreness lessens. Ice your feet after each stroll to reduce the inflammation. And to strengthen your arches, try this exercise. Place a towel flat on the floor and move it toward you by curling your toes. Repeat five times in each session. When this becomes too easy with practice, replace the towel with a book.

If the soreness in your arches continues despite these efforts, you may need custom arch supports or the attention of a medical professional.

Athlete's Foot

This itchy condition is the most frequent fungal infection of the skin. An athlete's foot infection frequently begins between the toes or on the soles of the feet. Walkers can become susceptible to the Trichophyton fungus when their feet sweat and their shoes are poorly ventilated. You can also pick up an infection when using public facilities such as locker rooms where the fungus sometimes thrives.

If you become infected, wash your feet daily and dry them carefully (particularly between the toes). A hairdryer works well for this. Consider purchasing socks made of fibers that wick moisture away from the skin. It is also wise to change your socks and shoes regularly, especially after walking. Antifungal creams can be purchased over the counter and usually can clear up symptoms within a few days. If one or more of your toenails has become infected, you will need to see a medical professional for treatment.

Blisters

The most common problem faced by walkers is blisters, which are caused by friction against the surface of the foot. A blister develops when two layers of the skin rub against each other and separate. To protect the inner skin, the body brings fluid to the area. One way to prevent this nuisance is by taking the time to get properly fitting shoes and socks. If the shoe itself is too tight or the sock makes it too snug, the skin can become irritated. Moisture also makes skin more susceptible to blistering, so consider purchasing walking socks that wick away moisture. Wearing two pairs of regular thin socks or placing a little petroleum jelly in the area where you anticipate a blister forming can also work as preventives.

As soon as you notice a burning sensation or a sore red spot somewhere on your foot, put a bandage there to avoid further irritation. For a small blister, apply an antiseptic to the area and cover it with moleskin or a bandage. A small blister is eventually likely to fall off naturally in the bath or shower. Larger blisters can be drained using a sterile needle, but do not remove the overlaying skin. Apply an antibiotic ointment and then place a bandage over the drained blister to promote healing.

Calluses

Sometimes a toughening of the skin occurs on the heel or ball of the foot because of friction or pressure. A small amount of this tough protective skin may not cause problems, but thicker calluses may become painful. Callused skin can be removed with a pumice stone to prevent such buildup. Soak the foot first in warm water, then rub the callus with the pumice stone. A callus pad can be placed around the callus to cushion it and ease pressure.

Corns

Corns are similar to calluses, but they occur on or between the toes. Sometimes these tough growths are painful. Tight shoes that put pressure on the toes are often the cause. The first step to relief is to start wearing shoes with a wider toe box (the front of the shoe where the toes reside).

To remove a corn, first soften the skin. Soak the foot in Epsom salt for fifteen minutes, then apply a moisturizer. Wrap the corn with moist gauze and then cover the foot with a secured plastic bag. After fifteen minutes, take off the bag and rub the corn with a pumice stone. Repeat this procedure once a day until the corn disappears. If the corn persists, see a podiatrist for treatment. Corn pads can be placed around the corn to make you more comfortable until it can be removed.

Heel Pain

One of the most common causes of heel pain can be plantar fasciitis. This condition is an irritation of the plantar fascia, a ligament that begins at the heel of the foot and continues forward to connect to bones in the front. The irritation is usually caused when the Achilles tendon or the calf muscles are too tight, and the plantar fascia is forced to stretch beyond its normal limits. This overstretching can also be caused by overpronation (too much inward rotation of the foot). Associated heel pain is noticed when sufferers first get out of bed in the morning or after a walk.

Stretching the calf muscles gently and slowly three times a day can help ease this problem. Icing the soles of your feet from the heel to the ball can be important after walking or when first rising from bed. It is smart to replace your walking shoes on a regular basis (after around 325 miles of use) to make sure your feet are adequately cushioned. Check your shoes now and see whether it's time to buy new ones. To provide sufficient support, the shoes should be bendable only at the forefoot and not at the center. Adding arch supports to your other shoes may be helpful too. Cutting back on your walking program may be necessary until the pain goes away. If these steps do not lessen the pain, see a medical professional.

Heel Spurs

A heel spur is a bony growth on the underside of the heel bone. It is usually an overuse injury, but it can also be caused by arthritis. Commonly, heel spurs are related to the condition known as plantar fasciitis we just discussed above. Sometimes with this condition, plantar fasciitis causes this ligament to tear and bleed. The bleeding may then lead to growths on the heel bone.

Icing the heel several times a day is recommended for heel spurs. Take a break from your walking routine until the pain subsides. When you return to activity, consider inserting foam cushions in the heels of your walking shoes for a time. If the pain continues, see a medical professional.

Ingrown Toenails

In this condition, the toenail grows into the flesh of the toe. The result can be pain, inflammation, and sometimes infection. Ingrown toenails can be the result of cutting the nail too short on the side, incurring an injury to the toe, or having an inherited tendency.

Ingrown toenails can sometimes be prevented by cutting the nail straight across. If you already have an ingrown nail, you may be able to retrain it to grow in a healthy way. First, soak the foot, then prop the nail away from the skin with sterile tweezers. Place a small amount of cotton under the nail to keep it from growing inward again.

Troublesome ingrown toenails may need professional medical treatment from a podiatrist.

Seasonal Clothing and Equipment

Clothing for walkers has three basic qualities: it is lightweight; it should fit loosely to allow room for movement; and it should be chosen based on your walking environment—be it warm or cold conditions, clear or rainy days, and day or nighttime. Here's a review of your various options.

Warm-Weather Clothing

Years ago, cotton was king in warm-weather sportswear. Today, many people are choosing synthetic fabrics or combination materials (natural fibers blended with synthetics) designed to keep you dry and cool during workouts in summerlike conditions. These soft, lightweight materials allow the skin to breathe. Such high-tech fabrics are a great choice, though they tend to be pricey. Natural fibers such as cotton may cost less and are a good second option.

The primary consideration in choosing warm-weather clothing is that it be loose fitting and offer breathability. Light colors (not black) will keep you cooler on hot days. A lightweight long-sleeved shirt can be worn at the beginning of your walk, then removed and tied to your waist as your body warms up. The shirt can be put back on if sunburn becomes a concern. Make sure the tops you choose do not restrict your arm movement. Bottoms, whether shorts, tights, or pants, should not have bulky interior seams that might cause chafing.

If you live in an extremely hot, sunny region or at high altitudes, you might consider purchasing "sun-protective clothing" that is made to block harmful UV rays that cause skin damage and even skin cancer.

Feet sweat more on hot days, and this can lead to blisters or a fungal infection. Consider using an antifungal powder during the hottest dog days of summer, and make sure your shoes are ventilated. Wear socks designed to wick sweat away from the skin.

You will be more motivated to keep walking if you protect your eyes from the glare of the sun, which can cause headaches and eyestrain. Hats, whether they are visors or cover the entire head, should provide adequate eye shielding. If you are balding, you will want to make sure the top of your head is covered to prevent sunburn. Choose a comfortable hat that fits properly so it will survive the entire walk. It should also be secure enough on your head that it will not blow off in the wind. As with your other articles of clothing, breathability is a factor in choosing the right hat.

Look for sunglasses that provide ultraviolet (UV) protection, as there is increasing evidence that long-term exposure to the sun causes eye damage. Consider only those glasses that offer 100 percent protection. Also think about the light conditions in the areas where you walk. If your route is regularly through the woods, you want glasses that let in more light. If you usually walk at the beach in the bright sun, the glasses you select should block more light. Purchase glasses only if they are a good, comfortable fit; you don't want them falling off your nose when you sweat.

Sunscreen should be used on all areas of your body that will be exposed. Purchase a product that offers a sun protection factor (SPF) of 50. (This number means that you will be able to stay outside fifty times longer than normal.) Use mineral based sunscreens that physically block the UV rays and look for higher percentage of zinc oxide and titanium dioxide which are more effective. Broad-spectrum UVA and UVB protection are both needed for full protection. Choose a sunscreen that is water-resistant for at least eighty minutes. A higher price doesn't mean better protection. Look at the expiration date. Apply the sunscreen at least fifteen minutes before you leave the house.

Wearing a cotton neckband or headband can offer relief to walkers on scorching summer days. You just dip the band in water and then wear it. The cotton bands are filled with water-absorbing gels and stay cool for hours.

On extremely hot days, it is best not to walk during midday when temperatures reach their highest and the sun is directly overhead. Drink water before and after your walk on hot days, and always take water along with you to sip during your stroll. In hot weather, fill up your water bottle one-half to three-quarters full and put it in the freezer overnight. This way, you will have cool, refreshing water for your entire walk the next day.

Cold-Weather Clothing

You don't have to hibernate during the winter months or when an unseasonable cold spell strikes. Nor do you need to weigh yourself down with heavy clothing when you go out for your walk. High-tech, lightweight fabrics can play a role in keeping you comfortable when the weather gets chilly. You will still want to dress in layers (a time-tested strategy for surviving cold weather), but now advanced fabrics allow the layers to be lighter. Tip: If you're unsure of how much clothing you will need to wear, it is better to err on the side of putting on too much. You can always remove something.

Start with a bottom layer that keeps you dry and warm, such as a turtleneck or crewneck top and long johns made of polyester or polypropylene. These lightweight, soft, high-tech materials will pull the sweat away from your body. Or try silk thermals, which are the natural version of the new synthetics. If it's not extremely cold, you may just need one layer of clothing on your legs. If that is the case, an outdoor pair of tights made of one of the high-performance fabrics is a good bet. The best ones have a brushed, soft interior surface.

For your middle layer, choose a material that will insulate you even when wet. A wool sweater is okay, but a fleece top or vest made of a high-tech fabric will be lighter. If you go with fleece, choose a top or vest that zips in the front so you can open it if you begin to feel too warm. If it is extremely cold, consider investing in a duck or goose down vest or a vest containing a battery pack that warms up the vest, similar to an electric blanket. For your legs, choose an unrestrictive pair of sweatpants made of a modern material such as Ultra-wick that can keep you comfortable and dry.

Your outer layer should be a jacket made of a windproof and waterproof material such as nylon or Gore-Tex. This will be important because wind gusts steal heat from your body. Hoods and pockets are useful features. And when the temperatures really drop or the wind is extreme, you can also wear pants made of the same material. Dark colors will keep you warmer.

Do not forget to protect your head, feet, hands, and neck in cold weather. A hat of wool or polyester will keep your head warm; look for one that covers your ears, perhaps with flaps. Fling a soft, synthetic fleece scarf around your neck. Socks made of wool or polyester will keep your feet comfortable. And wool or polyester mittens are preferable to gloves because your fingers can keep each other warm. Try a pair of mittens with a soft Primaloft fabric, a synthetic downlike material.

Footgear for slippery surfaces should have a heavier tread for a better grip. Outdoor clothing companies sell "snow sneakers," featuring knobby soles with traction. To use regular walking shoes in winter, you want a pair with knobs on the bottom that stick out at least three-eighths of an inch. Also look for a softer midsole (called "compression-molded EVA" in the shoe business) that will not get stiff in cold weather and will retain its cushioning ability.

Cold-weather walking can be exhilarating and a pleasant break from the overheated indoors. One trick is to walk into the wind on the way out so that it will be at your back on your return when you are more tired.

Rainy-Weather Clothing

Rain doesn't have to keep you indoors either. In fact, a walk in the rain can be a refreshing way to get back in touch with nature. Your senses come alive as you listen to the rain splash down, smell the moist earth, hear the excited birds sing (have you ever noticed how much birds warble when it rains?), and enjoy feeling secure and warm under your umbrella and/or poncho.

With a poncho, you will have plenty of room to maneuver, so much, in fact, that you could even fit a backpack under it. Ponchos are now available in synthetic materials that breathe, unlike the earlier rubber or plastic versions. An umbrella can double as a walking stick when the downpour is not threatening to soak you.

Nighttime Walking Clothing

To be more visible at night, try clothing made from high-tech materials that reflect light. Jackets, vests, tights, and water bottle holsters are all available in such glow-in-the-dark materials. Look for these items at sporting goods stores or in catalogs from outdoor equipment companies.

Other Assorted Gear

Here are a few more items that will add to your walking experience:

Earphones: You can use these if you choose music that creates a pleasant mood and keeps you walking. There are some excellent Zen meditations and relaxing music available.

Fanny pack: A small one can provide all the room you need to store such things as house keys, driver's license, some cash, and even your cell phone if you feel more secure bringing it. *Water bottle:* You might find one with its own netted cover and strap for easy carrying. You might experiment with different sizes to get a sense of how much water you will actually need. You do not want to carry too much; water is heavy.

All Dressed Up, So Get Going

When you are properly equipped, you will find that your walking program will run more smoothly. You will not be distracted in the middle of your walk because you did not think about bringing a water bottle, sunglasses, or your house keys. You will be able to focus on using the proper technique instead of worrying about what you don't have with you. When you select the right footgear, you will suffer from fewer foot problems and have less downtime. And having clothes for any type of weather you encounter can help you stay in shape no matter what the conditions are outside. Taking the time to gather the things you need will support your efforts and keep you on track.

Acknowledgments

There are many people whose guidance, support, and encouragement made this book possible.

We would like to thank our developmental editor, Rick Benzel, for his thoughtful assistance in putting together each of the chapters. We thank our literary agent, Jeff Herman, for his enthusiasm and commitment to seeing the importance and value of this book and helping to connect us to our publisher, Skyhorse. Our gratitude goes out to Skyhorse's executive editor, Daniela Rapp, for her championing of the book and shepherding it into fruition.

We thank our friends who read the manuscript, in whole or in parts, and provided helpful feedback: Albert Setton, Teresa Conrow, and Paula Dashiell.

We thank Margaret Phillips for the use of her beautiful garden for the videos and Wil Fernandez of FF Cinema for his expert cinematography. We thank Christopher Ruth for his technical support, as always.

Deep bows to our teachers who inspired us as we worked on the book: Thich Nhat Hanh, Trudy Goodman, Christian Wolf, Thich Thien An, Jean Pierre Marques, Share K. Lew, See Han Kim, Chapur Rinpoche, and Sun Shurong.

We thank all of our beloved Emperor's College colleagues and the Deepening Your Practice sangha at Insight LA.

Finally, we thank the Cassidy, Chu, Csintalan, Currie, Duterme, Fine, Fuller, Gerla Gustafson, Hirsh, Johnson, Kendrick, Kim, Krieger, Kunzelmann, Lee, Lugembe, Marques, Martino, MoraMarco, O'Connor, Paiar, Park, Pearson, Ristaino, Rosen, Setton, Vasquez, Weinstein, Zaidman, and Zhao families for their love and support.

About the Authors

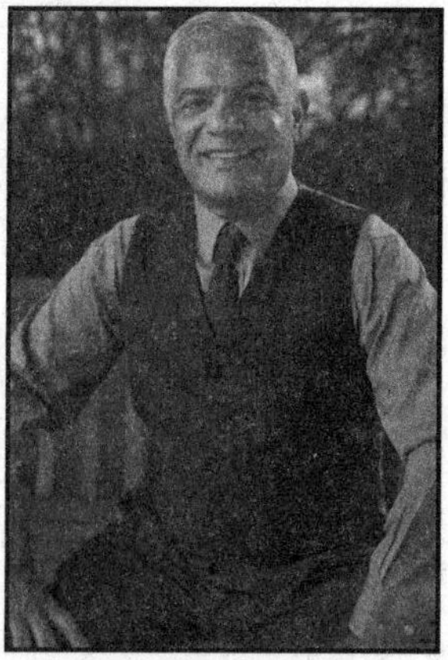

Jacques MoraMarco, a doctor of traditional East Asian medicine, is a licensed acupuncturist since 1977. He took the first acupuncture licensing examination ever administered in the state of California. He apprenticed with See Han Kim, a renowned teacher of traditional Korean medicine, who was trained monastically. He completed his postgraduate work at École Européene d'Acupuncture in Paris. From 1994 to 2004 he studied Sun tai chi with Sun Shurong in Beijing, China, and he is a fourth-generation lineage holder of Sun tai chi. He is a cofounder of the International Sun Tai Chi Association. Dr. MoraMarco is dean emeritus at the former Emperor's College of Traditional East Asian Medicine.

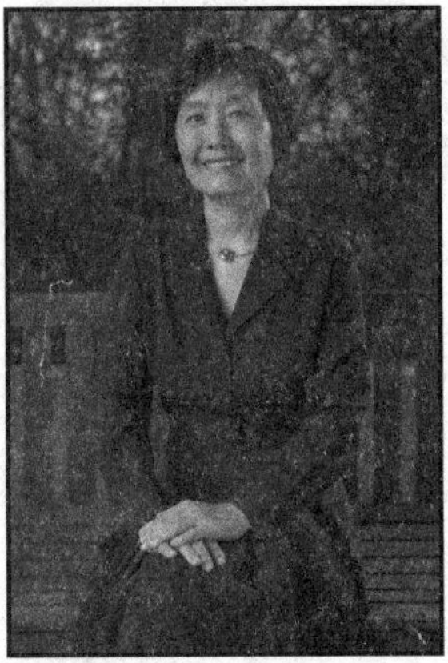

Yun Kim is the founder of Emperor's Wellness, a doctor of traditional East Asian medicine, a fifth-generation lineage holder of Sun tai chi, and has practiced mindful meditation for the past twenty years. A licensed acupuncturist in the state of California, she completed her doctoral clinical rotation at the PTSD clinic at the VA Greater Los Angeles Health System and maintains an acupuncture practice in Los Angeles. She earned her Doctor of Education at the University of Southern California, Rossier School of Education.

Notes

Week 1

1 American Heart Association, "Heart Disease Remains Leading Cause of Death as Key Health Risk Factors Continue to Rise," American Heart Association Newsroom, accessed August 1, 2025, https://newsroom.heart.org/news/heart-disease-remains-leading-cause-of-death-as-key-health-risk-factors-continue-to-rise.

2 "Walking for Health," Harvard Health, accessed August 1, 2025, https://www.health.harvard.edu/exercise-and-fitness/walking-for-health.

3 Julie Corliss, "Higher Step Counts Linked to Lower Risk of Heart-Related Death," Harvard Health, November 1, 2023, accessed August 1, 2025, https://www.health.harvard.edu/heart-health/higher-step-counts-linked-to-lower-risk-of-heart-related-death.

4 Maciej Banach et al., "The Association between Daily Step Count and AllCause and Cardiovascular Mortality: A MetaAnalysis," *European Journal of Preventive Cardiology* 30, no. 18 (2023): 1975–85, https://doi.org/10.1093/eurjpc/zwad229.

5 American Heart Association, "Walk This Way—It's Quite Good for You," American Heart Association News, April 1, 2024, accessed August 1, 2025, https://www.heart.org/en/news/2024/04/01/walk-this-way-its-quite-good-for-you.

6 Simon, S. (2017). Study: Even a Little Walking May Help You Live Longer. American Cancer Society. https://www.cancer.org/research/acs-research-news/study-even-a-little-walking-may-help-you-live-longer.html.

7 Sandee LaMotte, "Daily Walking May Slow Progression of Alzheimer's Disease, Study Finds," CNN Health, July 28, 2025, accessed August 1,

2025, https://www.cnn.com/2025/07/28/health/alzheimers-disease-walking-exercise-wellness.

8 Sandee LaMotte, "Walk This Number of Steps Each Day to Cut Your Risk of Dementia," CNN Health, September 6, 2022, accessed August 1, 2025, https://www.cnn.com/2022/09/06/ealth/steps-dementia-risk-wellness.

9 "Why You Should Move—Even Just a Little—Throughout the Day." Harvard Health, https://www.health.harvard.edu/heart-health/why-you-should-move-even-just-a-little-throughout-the-day.

10 Lee, M. et al., "Association of Step Volume and Intensity with All-Cause Mortality in Older Women," *JAMA Internal Medicine* 127, no. 8 (2019): 1105–212, https://doi.org /10.1001/jamainternmed.2019.0899.

11 Brage, S., Woodcock, J., Garcia, L. et al., "NonOccupational Physical Activity and Risk of Cardiovascular Disease, Cancer and Mortality: A DoseResponse MetaAnalysis of Large Prospective Studies, *British Journal of Sports Medicine* (2023): 1–15, https://doi.org/10.1136/bjsports-2022-105669.

12 Frost, Alexandra. "'Japanese Walking' Is a Great Way to Exercise, According to Experts." *The Washington Post*, July 13, 2025. https://www.washingtonpost.com/wellness/2025/07/13/japanese-walking-interval-walking-training/.

Week 2

1 Edouard Stiegler, *Régénération par la marche afghane* (Paris: Guy Trédaniel Editions, 2004).

Week 3

1 Maj van der Velden, A., et al. "Mindfulness Training Changes Brain Dynamics During Depressive Rumination: A Randomized Controlled Trial." *Biological Psychiatry* 93, no. 3 (2023): 233–242, https://doi.org / 10.1016/j.biopsych.2022.06.038.

Week 4

1 Qigong Institute, "EvidenceBase of Clinical Studies on QiGong: A Bibliometric Analysis," QigongInstitute.org, accessed August 1, 2025, https://www.qigonginstitute.org/abstract/15709/evidence-base-of-clinical-studies-on-qi-gong-a-bibliometric-analysis.

2 "Is More Exercise Always Better? Twin Study Challenges Longevity Myths," SciTechDaily, accessed August 1, 2025, https://scitechdaily.com/is-more-exercise-always-better-twin-study-challenges-longevity-myths.

3 American Cancer Society, "Exercise Linked with Lower Risk of 13 Types of Cancer," American Cancer Society Research News, accessed August 1, 2025, https://www.cancer.org/research/acs-research-news/exercise-linked-with-lower-risk-of-13-types-of-cancer.html.
4 Jones, B.M., "Changes in Cytokine Production in Healthy Subjects Practicing Guolin Qigong: A Pilot Study," *BMC Complementary and Alternative Medicine*, October 18, 2001, https://doi.org./10.1186/1472-6882-1-8.
5 Low, S. et al. (2024). Exploring Guolin Qigong (Mind-Body Exercise) for Improving Cancer Related Fatigue in Cancer Survivors: A Mixed Method Randomized Controlled Trial Protocol. *Integrative Cancer Therapies* (2024), https://doi.org/10.1177/15347354241252698.

Week 5

1 Wang, YangMing, "Inquiry on the Great Learning." ReligionOnline. Accessed August 1, 2025. https://www.religion-online.org/article/wang-yang-mings-inquiry-on-the-great-learning/.
2 "The Health Benefits of Tai Chi." Harvard Health, May 24, 2022. Accessed August 1, 2025. https://www.health.harvard.edu/staying-healthy/the-health-benefits-of-tai-chi.
3 Imoto, A. et al. (2021), "Evidence for the Efficacy of Tai Chi for Treating Rheumatoid Arthritis: An Overview of Systematic Reviews," *Sao Paulo Medical Journal* 139, no. 2 (2021); 91–97, https://doi.org/10.1590/1516-3180.2020.0346.R1.18112020.
4 Xinye Li, Peifen Chang, Min Wu et al., "Effect of Tai Chi vs Aerobic Exercise on Blood Pressure in Patients with Prehypertension: A Randomized Clinical Trial," *JAMA Network Open* 7, no. 2 (2024): e2354937, doi:10.1001/jamanetworkopen.2023.54937.
5 J. Zhao, J. P. C. Chau, A. W. K. Chan, Q. Meng, K. C. Choi, X. Xiang, Y. Zhao, R. He, and Q. Li, "Tailored Sitting Tai Chi Program for Subacute Stroke Survivors: A Randomized Controlled Trial," *Stroke* 53, no. 7 (2022): 2192–2203, https://doi.org/10.1161/STROKEAHA.121.036578.
6 Byeongsang Oh, et al.,"The Effects of Tai Chi and Qigong on Immune Responses: A Systematic Review and MetaAnalysis," Medicines 7, no. 7 (2020): 39, DOI: 10.3390/medicines7070039.
7 É. Cerqueira, D. A. Marinho, H. P. Neiva, and O. Lourenço, "Inflammatory Effects of High and Moderate Intensity Exercise—A Systematic Review," *Frontiers in Physiology* 10 (2019): 1550, https://doi.org/10.3389/fphys.2019.01550 (PubMed PMID 31992987; PMCID PMC6962351).

Week 7

1 Singh, B. et al., "Effectiveness of Physical Activity Interventions for Improving Depression, Anxiety and Distress: An Overview of Systematic Reviews," *British Journal of Sports Medicine* 57 (2023): 1203–9. https://bjsm.bmj.com/content/57/18/1203.

2 "Walking Fast Key to a Long Life? Study Links Pace to Aging," Study Finds, 2022. Accessed August 1, 2025. https://studyfinds.org/walking-faster-live-longer/.

Appendix A

1 Hirota Fujiki, Tatsuro Watanabe, Eisaburo Sueoka, Anchalee Rawangkan, and Masami Suganuma, "Cancer Prevention with Green Tea and Its Principal Constituent, EGCG: From Early Investigations to Current Focus on Human Cancer Stem Cells," *Molecules and Cells* 41, no. 2 (2018): 73–82, https://doi.org/10.14348/molcells.2018.2227 (PubMed PMID 29429153; PMCID PMC5824026).

2 Lenore Kohlmeier et al., "TransFatty Acid Levels and Breast Cancer Risk: A Case–Control Study," *Cancer Epidemiology, Biomarkers & Prevention*, September 1997 (UNC Chapel Hill press release), analyzing fat biopsies from 698 postmenopausal women and reporting a ~40 percent increased breast cancer risk for higher trans fatty acid levels.

3 Frank B. Hu et al., "Intake of Trans Unsaturated Fatty Acids and Risk of Coronary Heart Disease among Women," *New England Journal of Medicine* 337, no. 21 (1997): 1491–1499, doi:10.1056/NEJM199711203372102 (based on Nurses' Health Study data); Russell J. de Souza et al., "Intake of Saturated and Trans Unsaturated Fatty Acids and Risk of AllCause Mortality, Cardiovascular Disease, and Type 2 Diabetes: Systematic Review and MetaAnalysis of Observational Studies," *BMJ* 351 (2015): h3978, doi:10.1136/bmj.h3978.

Index

D

E

M

N

X

Y